PRAISE FOR
On Par

"The most humble and humane golf book I have ever read. Relying on insight instead of striving to incite, Pennington reduces golf to its most basic charms and makes the game remarkably accessible. Pennington has remarkably little ego and is the most noble of guides, encouraging and realistic, light and enlightening. Laid out like a challenging but attractive tract, *On Par* spares us the wiseguy tweaking with wisdom and earnest good humor. It should be handed to every first-time golfer as part of a welcome packet. Better yet, it should be in the zippered compartment of every new golf bag, like an in-flight magazine. Or a Bible." — ***New York Times Book Review***

"Golf writing may be unique among sportswriting for the way it often manages to convey the deadly seriousness those passionate about it feel toward the game, while simultaneously joking at their expense. Pennington's tone shares this trait and will be familiar to those who have read any of the many golf books out there. None of those books, however, offer nearly as much real-world advice to golfers on how to improve their experience. A must for beginning golfers or players looking to get more enjoyment out of their time on the course." — ***Kirkus Reviews***

"A hilarious, informative primer on the essentials of golf, schooling novices or the professional bewitched by mastering the links . . . . A chapter on golf-speak will tickle readers with a sampling of the colorful jargon of golf pros . . . With a few chuckles and basic instruction, Pennington's book effectively consolidates the wealth of knowledge from his beloved column, while delighting those who are perplexed by the puzzle that is the sport of golf." — ***Publishers Weekly***

On Par

THE EVERYDAY GOLFER'S SURVIVAL GUIDE

Bill Pennington

Mariner Books
Houghton Mifflin Harcourt
Boston • New York

First Mariner Books edition 2013
Copyright © 2012 by Bill Pennington
Illustrations © 2012 by Bob Eckstein

www.hmhbooks.com

Library of Congress Cataloging-in-Publication Data
Pennington, Bill, date.
On par: the everyday golfer's survival guide / Bill Pennington.
p. cm.
ISBN 978-0-547-54844-9 (hardback)   ISBN 978-0-544-00217-3 (pbk.)
1. Golf. I. Title.
GV965.P418 2012
796.352 — dc23
2011052072

Book design by Brian Moore

Printed in the United States of America
DOC 10 9 8 7 6 5 4 3 2 1

Portions of this book first appeared in the *New York Times* in different form.

To Joyce, Anne D., Elise, and Jack —
whatever the course, always the best partners

Contents

On Par

Introduction

They say golf is like life, but don't believe them.
Golf is more complicated than that.

GARDNER DICKINSON, longtime American tour pro

I BEGAN PLAYING golf seriously after college and was soon invited to an upscale private country club in Connecticut. As a former caddie, I knew how to dress the part and how to act, but my game was barely suitable for a dusty municipal course, let alone one of the more challenging layouts in the Northeast.

So, it was not a surprise that by the third hole I found myself in the deep rough a few feet behind a slender tree. I tried to chip out to the fairway but instead hammered my ball directly into the trunk of the tree before me. The ball ricocheted backward and struck me square in the forehead.

I hadn't hit the ball very hard, so I was mostly dazed by the impact. And, like many a beginner, I was frustrated. With an exasperated "That's unbelievable," I casually tossed the pitching wedge I was holding backward over my head. I didn't fling it; I just lofted it in the air.

The club lodged in the low-lying limbs of a pine tree about 10 feet off the ground.

Now, this was getting embarrassing.

Fortunately, my hosts at the club — nice people, but they were my elders and they certainly expected me to behave — were busy on the opposite side of the fairway looking for an errant shot in the woods.

No one had seen my clown act. I was alone and unnoticed on my side of the hole.

I quickly grabbed another club from my bag, and since the tree branch with the pitching wedge was almost close enough to touch, I tossed the second club at the wedge, hoping to knock it free.

If you play golf, you know what happened next. The second club caught in the tree, too.

Now, with great haste, I drove my golf cart under the tree limb and stood on the back of the cart so I could shake the branch with one hand as I smacked it with a third club held in my other hand. It was at this moment that the cart with my gracious hosts pulled up beside me.

And there I was, well dressed and well mannered, except I was standing on a golf cart using both hands to extricate not one but two of my golf clubs that had somehow ended up suspended in a tree.

I turned and tried to smile.

"What's that big red welt on your forehead?" one of my hosts asked.

"I hit myself with my ball," I answered.

You might wonder how an early golf day like that could have led to the next two decades of (mostly) happy golfing. I admit, at that moment, it's not what I would have predicted.

But then, I didn't expect my hosts to break out laughing. I didn't expect to laugh, too, trying to explain myself. And I did not expect them to then recount their own stories of golf misfortune, stories that might not have ended up with them shaking a tree for mislaid clubs but were nonetheless in the category of "the things this game will make you do."

So it was at that moment, perhaps for the first time, that I felt like a golfer.

Does being a golfer mean enduring clumsy embarrassment? Well, yes, it does sometimes, but that wasn't the point. Being a golfer is to join a tribe with an elaborate set of tenets and canons, one with its own mores and protocols and no definable mission other than to chase a little ball into a hole.

It is a silly game, somewhat childish, a good walk spoiled, as Mark Twain said. It is all those things. So why do we love this game?

The allure of golf is its simplicity, which leads to a thousand complexities. It is sophisticated because it is subtle. It is perfect because it is wholly and forever imperfect.

I once asked David Duval, the 2001 British Open champion, what makes golf so difficult and yet so appealing. He said, "It's all the time to think between shots."

I asked the great Phil Mickelson the same question and he said, "It's all the choices you have."

I asked Jack Nicklaus and he replied, "Because you must master so many elements, including yourself."

I asked the golf commentator and author David Feherty and he said, "Because it's a ridiculous game and it's our fault for playing it."

I was tempted to ask Feherty if he had ever lost two clubs in a tree on one hole but realized it wasn't necessary. He would understand.

This is a book that speaks to both the exultant and troubled souls of golfers everywhere, men and women like me who are transfixed by the game and long to understand it. Golf is an endeavor of hope, fear, disappointment, glee, perseverance, abandonment, unrelenting gratification and unexpected reward, certain punishment, integrity, cheating, camaraderie, isolation, technology, and oneness with nature, all governed by a stifling set of ancient rules frequently undone by an unseen yet officially recognized karma called "rub of the green."

We, the golf tribe, take our golf with eyes wide open — the better to let tears of frustration and of joy flow freely.

I have played golf seriously for the last thirty years and have covered and written about the game throughout that time as well. For the last several years, I have written a weekly golf column in *The New York Times* called "On Par," which has let me come face-to-face with all the simplicities and complexities of golf in its many arenas. But newspaper columns are brief. A book allows us to examine golf's length and breadth, to propose and ponder solutions to the seemingly unsolvable. Because golf is much more than the quest to master the actual game. Golf transports the player to a foreign land and culture with its own set of mores and protocols. It is a world with quizzical and ever-changing weaponry and settings of great beauty but treacherous hazards.

Golf is often likened to a battle of self, a crucible of temptation and honor, and it is, but even that seems an understatement since golf means learning to deal with maddening playing partners, changing weather conditions, astonishing inequities, and ugly clothes, not the least of which is hopelessly goofy shoes.

Then there are the basic steps of learning the game and the behemoth of golf instruction. Everything about this helpful community of teachers is inherently confusing, which might explain why there are several hundred theories on the correct way to learn golf and another thousand theories on how to get better at it. The reality is that the golfing indoctrination never truly ends. The game even has its own ever-evolving language.

And yet, there is no more dedicated tribe than golfers. If they are not exactly the definition of contentment, they are hearty and resolute. If love means never having to say you're sorry, then golf means never having to say you're satisfied.

Why do golfers say that it never rains on the golf course? Because even when it does, there is nowhere else they would rather be. Why do few serious golfers quit the game? Because they are convinced they are one keen golf tip, or one discerning golf book, away from learning the secret to good golf for good. Why do presidents of the United States play golf? Because it makes running the free world seem easy.

In the pages that follow, I will lead every golfer on the path to golf fulfillment. Do you believe that?

No? Thank goodness, because there is no fulfillment in golf. We might treat it like one but golf is not a religion; it is a game. However, there are golf canons and principles. There is golf enlightenment and golf secrets, too. There are golf commandments. There are saints, or at least really nice, helpful people. There are golf gods. There is a golf promised land, if not many promised lands. And there is surely golf hell, again, in multiple forms.

But perhaps most central to being a golfer is something truly indispensable: the belief, even the conviction, that you will get better.

Just as fundamental: the ability to distort reality so you will likely get better or at least have fun trying.

Let's examine each.

1. The belief or conviction that you will get better

Golf is so routinely humiliating that if we didn't know we were going to improve, it's doubtful we could press on. "One of the real truths about golf is that even the best players in the world sometimes shake with terror and wonder if they will ever hit the ball straight again in their entire life," Lee Trevino said. "I'm serious. I've stood over the ball and prayed that the clubface would find the ball at all. It's the loneliest feeling in the world."

Annika Sorenstam once told me she wondered — in the middle of several competitive rounds — if she could get the ball airborne. "I would hit a couple of shots that just squirted away across the ground," she said. "As a professional, you would think those shots would never happen again, but they do. I took whatever club I thought would get the ball anywhere up in the air. That was my entire goal. I think it was a 7-iron. It wasn't the right club to reach the green; I just wanted to see the ball in the air for a change."

But in these dark depths, even the best players, who in struggling moments like these have fallen farther and lost far more touch than the average beleaguered player, nonetheless were resolute in their belief that they would get better.

"I feel sorry for the people who give up golf because it's too hard," Trevino said. "They miss the exhilaration of getting it right, even if for just an hour or a day or week. And that exhilaration is not just watching the physical turnaround, like the ball soaring in the sky and dancing on the green. They miss the feeling of knowing they refused to give up and hung in there long enough to make the turnaround happen. That's golf, too, proving you can do it."

Said Sorenstam: "People say golf is unforgiving but it's not. Golf can be unkind, yes, but golf rewards those who persevere. If you stick with it, when you might least suspect it, golf can suddenly be very generous. Does any golfer really think that eighteenth-hole birdie or that last beautiful drive or iron shot is an accident? How often after your worst holes do you play your best golf? Golf has mercy."

It is the nature of all golfers to believe the elusive secret of golf awaits around the next dogleg. That's not true, but some clues to the secret unquestionably lie in our path every time we pick up a club. Because great shots can and do appear like magic, golfers are imbued early on with the sense that the same magic lingers on the golf course — eager to return on the same whim with which it exited. Which is, in fact, likely. That is the happenstance part of golf, which is more real than it may sound.

But it is also an elemental truth for every golfer that he or she has executed several, probably hundreds, of indisputably great golf shots. That is the basis for the steadfast conviction that we will all get better. The experience, sensation, and impression of a good shot are so primitively nourishing that all bad shots, however unremitting, turn into annoying but seemingly unrelated interludes — nothing more than long pauses between good shots.

That is golf.

2. The ability to distort reality so you will likely get better or at least have fun trying

I once surveyed dozens of top golf teachers on an unusual subject: What does the typical everyday recreational golfer do well?

We talk about what we do wrong all the time, so I was wondering what we do right, you know, what are we good at?

The first thing golf pros mentioned was how good a game average golfers talk after a round. Which is another way of saying we talk about our good shots and purge from memory most of the bad ones.

"The most endearing thing about the average golfer is the ability to see the good in a shot that may not have brought a good result," John Elliott Jr., a top-ranked teacher, said. "People say, 'I hit it good; it was just a bad lie.' Or 'It was heading right for the fairway until it hit that little tree limb.'

"In fact, they probably shouldn't have hit it anywhere near that tree but they see the positive. Average golfers think they are far better than they really are. And that's really important because golf is a hard game and you need confidence or you're sunk. Average golfers seem to get this instinctively. Listen to them at the nineteenth hole. Their golf games are just great there."

This is no random observation. Another top teacher, Don Hurter, who is based near Denver, said a golfer who lacks the capacity to over-rate his or her game rarely progresses.

"I see it with promising junior golfers," Hurter said. "Everybody plays badly some of the time, but the golfers who see their mistakes more than their accomplishments end up finding this game just too hard to enjoy. Some of the best golfers in the history of the game almost went out of their way to find excuses for bad shots."

It is said that Jack Nicklaus in his prime would have a rationale for any shot that did not succeed exactly as planned. The rationale never came around to Nicklaus having a moment of ineptitude.

"I stood next to Jack during tournaments and watched him out-and-out shank the ball out-of-bounds," Dave Anderson, the Pulitzer Prize–winning sportswriter, told me years ago. "But when I asked him about it afterward, he would say, 'Well, actually I was trying to cut the ball left to right and it was a little on a side hill and I just overdid it and it went too left-to-right.' Or he might say the lie was bad and he was trying something else risky.

"I wanted to say, 'Jack, I was there. You just missed it — you hit it on the hosel of the club.' But I knew that in his mind, he always had a good plan and sometimes it just didn't work out. In his mind, there were rarely truly awful shots, just awful outcomes."

There is power in this way of thinking, and successful, happy golfers use it all the time. It's a philosophy that spills over into how we play. Why do we have scramble tournaments? So many poor shots won't count. Same thing in match play, and in many gambling games, like skins games or Nassaus. Lose the front nine? You can make up for it on the back nine. You can double bets when down two holes. Hit it into the bunker? So what? Get up and down in two and you win money for a sandie.

We rationalize the difficulties of golf in so many ways because we must.

Sean Foley, a Canadian pro who teaches in Florida and who has tutored many PGA Tour pros including Tiger Woods, tells many of his recreational students to ignore the scorecard altogether.

"People focus on the course rated par," Foley said. "That's a number set for what a pro is supposed to shoot. I tell my students, 'Today, the first hole isn't a par 4 like it says on the scorecard, it's a par 6. And the next hole isn't a par 5, it's a par 7.'

"So you know what happens? Some guy makes a 5 on the first hole and instead of feeling like a failure who made bogey, he strides to the next tee feeling great because he made birdie. Next hole he makes a par-saving putt for a 7 and again he feels good. That gets him confident and pumped up and you know what? He starts slamming the ball right down the middle because he's swinging easy and self-assured instead of tense and disappointed. He starts making real pars — 4s and 3s — because his frame of mind is positive.

"That's a real experiment that I've tried a hundred times and it works almost every time. It improves every level of golfer."

It is not really about distorting reality; it's about creating a new one.

Most golfers should practice this kind of mental gymnastics. Yes, you hit a 100-yard wedge poorly and left yourself 35 feet from the hole, but you're still putting for birdie. Yes, you missed the green altogether, but it's a chance to prove that your chipping practice in the backyard will pay off. Yes, you hit one into the woods, but hey, maybe you'll find some lost golf balls. OK, it's your fourth time in the woods today and you don't need any more dirty, muddy found golf balls. But look at it this way: You haven't had to reapply the sunscreen.

It is in this spirit of kinship that I give you the following chapters, which are meant not only to examine and illuminate golf in all its variety, but to make sure no golfer ever wanders alone. Golf's perplexities and befuddlements are our strength, our badge of honor. We share them, and this book embraces them.

I have played golf with Tiger Woods, hit balls with Trevino, been schooled in the game by Sorenstam. I have also played golf with people named Scooter, Lulu, and Hopsy, folks I ran into during an idle Thursday afternoon playing a quick nine holes. You can learn a lot playing golf with someone named Hopsy, or Tiger. And like the ebb and flow of eighteen holes, it is all about the journey. In the succeeding pages, let me tell you what I have learned. It will make you laugh and I promise it won't hurt. Or at least not too much.

Speaking of things that sting, three years and many golf lessons after my initial outing at that swanky private Connecticut club, I was invited back to play the course again. I would like to say that I birdied that third hole where I had my misadventure in the trees, but golf is a game of integrity, so I won't fib. My hosts were the same as they had been years earlier, and we spent several minutes laughing our way down the third fairway recalling our previous visit.

But there's the news. I was in the fairway.

Still, standing there, I absent-mindedly rubbed my forehead. What a game.

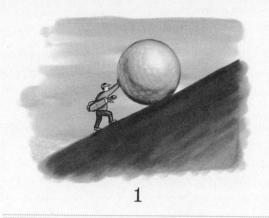

1

Essential Golf

The only thing a golfer needs is more daylight.

BEN HOGAN

GOLF WAS INVENTED by a bunch of bored Scottish sheep-herders. Little did they know that their invention would lead us 550 years later to the Technasonic golf ball measurer. What's the Technasonic? It's a little portable contrivance that weighs your golf ball and finds its exact equator so you can mark that spot with a felt-tip pen. Then, after teeing up your ball, all you have to do is hit that exact spot over and over to make the ball travel straighter and farther. Because, as we all know, if a golf ball's true equator could actually be identified, average golfers could always hit that spot. We would never miss it.

Why in God's name didn't somebody tell us about this magic equator spot before?

The Technasonic is a golf gadget that thousands of golfers believe they need and will routinely use. It is one of the hundreds of foolish golf devices that real golfers have no use for. Only pretend golfers have a Technasonic. Don't be a pretend golfer.

Golf is not a simple game. But we need not make it more complicated with things like the Technasonic. We need not make it more complicated with things like overly fancy head covers for our clubs or little clamps on the sides of our golf bags where the putter can be snapped into place to keep it from getting mixed up with all the other clubs.

Those little putter clamps actually deprive average golfers of one of the game's most important emotional releases: slamming the putter back into the bag after a missed 3-foot putt. So don't get one of those little clamps. You'll have to slam something else, like your hand, which might break, or you might try to kick your bag, which isn't advised either since it looks cowardly.

No, a putter aggressively thrust into a padded sleeve of the golf bag is one of the safest things you can do. (Especially if done when no one is looking.)

Being a golfer means understanding all these little nuances of the game. It would be much easier if golf were just about the act of playing the game, like Ping-Pong, where anything goes. You can play Ping-Pong barefoot and in your underwear with the lampshade from last night's Mojito party still on your head and a frying pan for a paddle. No one really cares. It probably won't affect your game either. Unless your opponent has a bigger frying pan. Essentially, in Ping-Pong, it doesn't matter how you dress, it doesn't matter what brand of ball you play, and it certainly doesn't matter if your shadow is interfering with your opponent's next shot.

But golf is not Ping-Pong — thank goodness — and in golf all those things matter to some degree. In golf, you will have to wear pants, shorts, skorts, or skirts, and someone might be counting the number of pockets adorning those garments. You will be expected to play at a certain pace. You will be assigned random gardening-like chores on the golf course, and you must at times acquire the stock-still stance of a Queen's Guard or be the target of angry stares and muttered grousing.

Sometimes it will seem as if every little thing matters in golf, and that's your cue that you are finally figuring out the game. It's also usually the point when someone else tells you that what you need to do is forget all the little things and just play.

"Relax, dude, it's just a game," your buddy will say after your third consecutive double bogey.

You will want to scream, shouting to one and all about how you could relax if only your head weren't filled with five new swing tips, if your designer golf belt weren't so tight, if your $200 gap wedge didn't hate you, and if the last three putts hadn't lipped out. But you will not scream or shout. You will instead do what all real golfers do at times like these. When your buddy isn't looking, you will slam your putter in your bag.

Now, the path to this golf enlightenment — not fulfillment, mind you, but enlightenment — has many steps. First, you must understand the true essentials of playing golf. In other words, if you're going to enter the belly of the beast, if you're going to be a golfer, what are the essential things you need and need to know? This is no minor thing. The average golfer spends about $600 a year on his or her golf game, and that's not counting greens fees. The average beginning golfer spends more than twice that, about $1,350, during the first year of playing the game. So this isn't trivial.

Let's start by debunking some myths. Here, for example, are the three most overrated golf essentials: tees, the golf bag, and everything someone else tells you on the golf course.

People actually pay money for tees, which are no more than little pieces of wood or plastic. I have never understood this. Keep your head down after you tee off (not a bad idea in general) and you will find so many discarded, perfectly good tees you won't be able to keep all of them in one golf bag.

But people think tees are important. Well, some people. Did you know that lots of British golfers don't even use tees? It is perfectly legal to smack the ground on the tee box with your club, raising a little tuft of grass that will form a mound that makes a perfect tee. Place the ball on that mound. If you are a golfer with a certain type of swing fault — like an open clubface at impact — the mound might even straighten out the face of your club and help you hit the ball straighter. In fact, until late in the nineteenth century, when the first tee was devised and patented, making a mound with their club or their hands was how all golfers began every hole.

Now, it is understandable that some people find solace in the look of a ball resting on a tee. It does usually breed confidence — who couldn't hit a ball perched in the air? And, with modern drivers that resemble a grapefruit pierced with a stick, it is necessary to get the ball teed up at least a few inches off the ground. This helps the launch angle characteristics of some drivers as well.

So in that case, we need tees, including a few 4-inch tees for our drivers. Again, you will find these on the ground, too. Plus, many golf courses, particularly resorts or private clubs, give them away in the pro shop.

But if you are a beginner or have lost your old golf bag or just feel the desire to buy some tees, when you go to the store or go online to purchase some, you're going to discover that the seemingly simple world of the golf tee has gone high-tech and — like so much else in golf — has gotten highly complicated.

There are now hundreds of kinds of tees made. There are tees designed to better the environment and tees made to better your breath (seriously). There are personalized tees, unbreakable tees, biodegradable tees made of cornstarch, pronged tees, and brush tees, with thin bristles like those on a toothbrush that hold up the ball.

Lest you think this is some kind of alternative niche golf spinoff, consider this: The United States Golf Association, which authorizes tees as conforming or not conforming to the Rules of Golf, commonly receives sixty new tee design applications annually. An Internet search of the United States Patent Office archives for golf tee patents returned a list of 1,298 since 1976.

More than 1.5 billion tees are sold globally every year. If that seems high, do a little math. There were about 500 million golf rounds played in the United States alone last year. A third of those rounds were only nine holes, so that adds up to about 8 billion holes played in the United States. That's a lot of broken or lost golf tees. And a big business.

Never mind that you could use a thimble, a AAA battery, or a plastic shot glass to tee up your golf ball and probably play just fine. The problem is that those things are household items, and like the old wooden golf tee, they aren't technologically advanced. And since we have technologically advanced drivers, hybrids, irons, putters, and golf balls, it figured we would soon have to have technologically advanced golf tees. And that's at the crux of the golf tee brand boom. The new devices, of course, promise to help you hit the ball farther and straighter.

Take the Zero Friction tee, which has three prongs that hold up the ball instead of the little concave cup atop a traditional golf tee. Golfers using this tee will gain 4 yards of distance and 5 yards of accuracy, the company contends, because its tee reduces contact between the ball and the tee.

"With our tee, you hit more pure ball and significantly less tee," John R. Iacono, the founder of Excel Golf Company, which makes the Zero Friction tee, told me. Iacono said his golf company had revenues of $5 million in 2009.

Iacono said Excel Golf had independent testing to back up its claims of distance and accuracy gains. Throughout the tee industry, there are companies that boast of test results showing the gains an alternative tee can produce. There is the Launcher tee, which has a 36 percent smaller "ball nest" and cites evidence that drives travel 8 yards farther and 50 percent straighter. The Stinger tee also has a smaller area upon which to rest the ball. Its proposed distance gain? Fourteen yards.

I have tried most of these tees. They are undeniably more durable because they are made of modern composites. It's hard to tell if they help you hit the ball any straighter or farther. A repeatable swing would help with the experiment; let me know if you find one.

At the USGA, they have the robots and machinery to validate or reject the claims of manufacturers. But the USGA does not release the findings of those tests. They do test the tees to see if they conform to the Rules of Golf. And what does the rule book say about tees? Not much.

A tee must not be bigger than 4 inches and must not be designed to help with the line of play. In other words, it can't have an arrow or pointer attached, and it must not be designed to "influence the movement of the ball."

What does that last part mean?

A general interpretation would be that the tee can't help a golfer hit the ball farther or straighter. Dick Rugge, the senior technical director of the USGA Test Center, said that about 80 percent of the tees sent to his office, including tees like the Zero Friction and the Launcher, are assessed as conforming to the Rules of Golf. Rugge wouldn't say much more than that. Asked if that meant these new tees helped players hit the ball farther, Rugge answered, "Our testing finds they don't influence the movement of the ball."

Hear the inference being screamed in that sentence?

Now there are tees sold, and used by a very few recreational golfers, that will influence the movement of the ball, mostly by helping to cure a slice or hook. These tees have a little half-sphere attached to the top that rests on the ball. The half-sphere takes much of the nasty sidespin off the ball that your open or closed clubface puts there at impact. These tees do not conform to the rules. They are illegal in competition.

You don't see many golfers using them because you might as well throw the ball down the fairway.

The biggest problem with alternative tees is the cost. Some sell for $3 to $4 each. Other tees, like the Zero Friction tee, cost considerably less, with a package of thirty-five or fifty retailing for about $7.

Now as I said, personally, I don't think I've bought a tee in twenty years. And I certainly would never pay more than a dime per tee. I have found plenty of the alternative tees and I use them. And if you buy alternative tees that you truly believe let you hit the ball farther, I'm not going to argue with you. Some players on the PGA Tour use them. Confidence is everything in golf. If you believe it works, it probably does.

But be mindful of the science and USGA testing. It's a myth that you need fancy tees. You do need some long tees for your driver. You can find them, in all colors, on the ground near most any tee box.

Once, I was at a clinic John Daly was giving, and the moderator asked him for a secret to his prodigious distance off the tee. Daly explained that before he hits, he always leans the tee forward so that it and the ball are tilting toward the target in the fairway.

"Really," the moderator said. "And how much distance does that add?"

Answered Daly: "About an inch."

So, what's the second most overrated golf essential?

The golf bag.

Ever seen these guys walking around the golf course carrying their clubs in what looks like an archer's quiver or an oversize holster? It has canvas sides, a single strap, and two small pouches for balls and other stuff (like found tees).

Ever notice that these guys are often good players?

Sometimes good golf comes down to eliminating the superfluous. Truth be told, if physically able, all golfers should walk more often when they play. It's good for you and studies show you will score better (more on that in a later chapter). One way to make it easier to walk is to have a tidy, small walking bag, something that's easy to sling over your shoulder after 90 — OK, 120 — shots during a round.

This doesn't mean it has to be unappealing. There are dozens of stylish golf bags weighing less than five pounds now made by manufacturers like Ogio, Sun Mountain, and all of the major golf companies: Titleist, Adidas, Callaway, TaylorMade, and Nike. All have kickstands.

So that's step one. Get a lightweight bag for hoofing it, or for practice sessions. Or just because a big golf bag is overrated and unnecessary.

I know what you are thinking: What about those fancy member-guest tournaments? Won't a lightweight bag make me look like a lightweight? Don't you need a big golf bag — known as a cart bag — for those occasions? Nobody wants to look cheesy.

Actually, so long as it isn't faded, stained, or spattered with mud, a small, trim bag will probably be welcome in most settings nowadays. Not only that, if you're going to be accompanied by a caddy, it will be warmly welcomed. You shouldn't ask a caddy to lug around a big cart bag.

Yes, every country club golfer once had a bag so hefty it barely fit in the trunk of that golfer's hefty Cadillac. But the typical Cadillac isn't as hefty as it once was, and neither is the typical golf bag. In some elite golf circles, you may need an additional, bigger cart bag for certain select occasions. For 90 percent of us, a new golf bag is a $150 purchase made once every two or three years, and it should not take more than thirty minutes out of our busy lives to choose one. And always consider downsizing.

Overrated as it may be, there are still a few essentials to a good golf bag. It must have a separate waterproof compartment for your valuables, such as your cell phone (turned off, of course), your wallet or small purse, jewelry, keys, or money. Waterproof is key. You need at least one full-length apparel pocket to house a rain jacket or sweater. It has to be big enough to contain two garments and an extra towel. It does not have to be big enough to hide a small load of laundry.

Only professional golfers need that kind of space. Hall of Famer Annika Sorenstam was once in the middle of an LPGA tournament round when she asked her caddie to get something out of her bag. But just as he reached for that zipped pocket, she remembered something and yelped, "No, not that pocket."

But it was too late. One zip and out tumbled Sorenstam's dirty laundry all over the fairway. Fans watching laughed. As did Annika, though she quickly started stuffing laundry back into the bag.

It seems that morning, Annika had been in a hurry packing at her hotel, and as she was heading out the door, she glanced at the bathroom and saw that she had forgotten a pile of already worn clothes in the bathroom. With her suitcases already packed, she stuffed the clothes in her golf bag.

"That's not one of my usual golf lessons for average golfers," she told me. "In fact, don't do that. As pros, our bags are so big because it means the names of our sponsors will be bigger and more visible. We don't really need all this room either.

"Well, maybe that day I did."

But you do need a pocket on the outside of the golf bag to store your golf balls. After you've plunked one—OK, two—balls into a pond, and there's steam rising out of your ears, you don't need the added frustration of wrestling with the various pockets of your bag, looking for another ball. Make sure that pocket is easily accessible and user-friendly. Many now use magnetic closures instead of zippers to ease the irritation.

You will also need a double-strap carrying system and something soft, like fleece, at the top of the dividers that separate the clubs on the interior of the bag so that the shafts of your clubs are protected. It's nice to have an easily reached pocket for a drink or bottle of water. Everything else is optional, and don't choose too many options. You don't need a special flat, scorecard-holding slot or an extra ball clasp where balls snap into place.

One way to think of your golf bag is as a reflection of your golf personality. Do you want it to be loud and showy? Do you want it to be colossal and bigger than life, making you look like a high-maintenance golf course personality? Do you want your bag to have lots of moving parts, or do you want it to be like a good golf swing — simple and efficient? How do you want your bag to arrive at the first tee? With a look-at-me thud? Or noiselessly, gently settling in the grass, calm and confident? Do you want it adorned with all those extra balls affixed to the outside, something that shouts, "Look how many balls are going to be needed today!"?

Or do you want it to be austere, with a look of confident discretion that states, "Today, I'm going to take out one ball, and only one ball."

The basics of the golf bag are basic. Keep it clean and pick a color or a pattern that makes you smile. You will need the unspoken encouragement out there. So make it simple. Golf is complicated enough.

Here is my last overrated or presumed essential: everything one of your friends or your favorite uncle the good golfer has ever told you.

In the words of Butch Harmon, former coach to Tiger Woods and Greg Norman and the longtime tutor to Phil Mickelson: "More bad golf habits are learned trying to listen to somebody else's tips on the game. Unless you have exactly the same build, the same athleticism, the same flexibility, the same personality, the same clubs, and the same golf goals, taking advice from another golfer is the surest way to get worse at golf. You might as well throw all your clubs in a pond or run them over with your car.

"What works for another golfer will almost never work for you."

How's that for making it plain?

But you don't have to take Butch's word for it. You can prove it yourself.

Have you ever played in a scramble where everyone plays a ball from the same spot, trying to hit a shot on the green or sink a putt? As each person hits, the other golfers stand behind that player, and what you see is that almost all of the players, even the good ones, line up their club or putter differently. They aim at different spots, even if the hole is only 4 feet away. They rarely actually aim at the hole or the green.

When the swing begins, each golfer's club usually takes a different path to the ball, and the shaft is angled sometimes in exotic ways. Arms, hips, shoulders, and hands are all moving and thrashing in so many directions. You will notice that everyone swings with different rhythms, and everyone contacts the ball at different places on the clubface.

Some golfers hit balls left to right or right to left or straight. Some swings are steep and some are shallow. Some people take big divots of dirt and some pick the ball clean off the turf. Some shift their weight foot to foot and some do not.

There are almost as many ways to play golf as there are players.

And yet, we recreational golfers routinely let strangers we may have met just an hour earlier tell us how to play golf.

"Hey, your grip is a little weak," someone will say just after he's struck a good shot and you haven't. "You should try using my grip. It's stronger."

And that's how you'll hold the club perhaps for the next three years. All kinds of things might be going wrong and you might try a hundred fixes. But all along, it could be your grip that's the problem, and it's something you picked up on a whim one day.

"In every other part of their life, people are careful who they take advice from," Jim McLean, named one of America's top five golf teachers by *Golf Digest,* said to me once. "They don't let just anyone advise them on their finances. They won't let a buddy tell them how to raise their kids or which house to buy. People understand that whether it's what clothes they wear or what food they like to eat, it's a personal thing.

"But when it comes to golf, if someone hits a few good shots during a round, it's like, 'Hey, how did you hit that?' One guy might be 6-4 and 220 pounds and the other might be 5-8 and 150 pounds. They can't exchange golf swings any more than they can exchange golf shirts."

But people do it. For instance, have you witnessed this scene?

Three guys are talking in the bar after a round. One guy gets off his barstool and starts demonstrating a certain swing move or the way to hit some shot.

Next thing you know, all three of them are standing near the bar, practicing this maneuver.

The next time you see this scene, I have my own advice. Try to join those guys the next time they are playing, making it a foursome. It will be a fantastic chance to win some money because all three of them will be all screwed up for weeks.

Now, of course, the point is not that you always have to go it alone on the golf course. It's part of the fun to compare notes and strategies. But choose your golf instruction oracles carefully. A certified PGA professional is a good place to start, and you can probably get a series of five group lessons for $100 if you have not taken lessons before. Along the way you can find a teacher with whom you have a rapport or with whom you feel you can develop one. And don't keep going to that teaching pro if you see no progress. Find another one. There are more than 28,000 nationwide.

At the same time, obviously, it's fun to read game-improvement tips in magazines, but they are offered by pros, too, not your uncle or one of your friends. Learn what works for you. I've often thought it was a good idea to read the tips and instruction from only one golf magazine and not several. I read both *Golf* and *Golf Digest,* for example, but I read the instruction articles from only one or the other in any given year because I find that the two magazines contradict each other on a regular basis. This game is hard enough without having to sort out whom to believe every month.

In the end, however, you probably do need to seek out some kind of expert counsel. This is especially true for beginning golfers, they of the $1,350 in spending during that first, overexcited year when they are bitten by the golf bug. Beginners often feel as if they've suddenly joined a mysterious cult and they are most susceptible to unhelpful, misguided advice.

Suzy Whaley, a popular Connecticut golf teacher and a member of the PGA of America's national instruction committee, notes that beginners do need to know how to hold the club, how to stand to the ball, how to maneuver around the golf course, and how to use the different clubs to get the ball in the hole. And an instructor can teach all that and can be that early golfing buddy who assuages the pressure beginners feel to perform well immediately in what, to them, is an alien environment.

"The notion that golf is brutally hard prevents a lot of people from ever playing," said Whaley, one of the very few women to qualify and play in a PGA Tour event. "I tell people that you don't have to be great to have fun at it. We will help you get the ball in the air, and you'll enjoy the time out there with your spouse, friends, or children."

Among Whaley's recommendations is that new golfers not begin at the tee box but instead drop a ball 150 yards from the hole and play in from there.

"You still get all the elements of golf, and you don't have to feel the pressure to keep up," she said. "When you can make double par — an 8 on a par 4 — move back to 200 yards away. And when you can make double par from there, move back to the family tee box or some other forward box. And so on."

Those are good tips worth heeding. As for the others you might hear out on the golf course, it's all right to listen. Be polite because no harm is meant. But when the advice is over, just smile and ignore it.

OK, if there are overrated essentials, then there must be underrated ones, right?

And there are. Let's start, for example, with good practice balls. It is my belief that most golfers don't really learn how to play the game at the golf course but in the backyard. Some people think they learn at the driving range, and they could if they did many things differently at the range. More on that later. But most golfers ignore the gains that can be had in the backyard. It's the perfect golf laboratory for golfers of all ability levels, provided you have a backyard (you don't need more than 30 yards). You can sometimes get some of the same work done hitting into a net.

It is in the backyard that you can hone your pitching and chipping.

It is in the backyard that you can build a repeatable swing. It is in the backyard that you can learn to shape the ball, hitting fades and draws. It is in the backyard that you can learn self-control when you cannot seem to do any of these things with any proficiency.

Or, you can learn what happens if you don't have self-control. I still have the pitching wedge I wrapped around a backyard tree. And so, it is in the backyard that you can also amuse your neighbors.

But the key is good practice golf balls. There are a lot of types of practice golf balls because they have been around for decades. Some are pretty useless, like the hard white plastic ones with no holes. They do not mimic a true ball's flight in any way. But in recent years companies have designed far superior alternatives. One of the best is the BirdieBall, which reacts off the club head like a real ball but flies no more than 40 yards and lands softly. It won't break windows either, which is an important consideration.

The BirdieBall looks like a napkin ring or hair curler, but it's tough plastic and the aerodynamics give it the real-ball feel off the club. And you can also purchase a distinctive hitting mat called the StrikePad. The StrikePad is different in that it isn't flat like a traditional hitting mat but is instead cambered, so it absorbs more of the shock of a downward iron swing. It is also lightweight so you can move it around the backyard and hit down on shots without taking a divot out of your lawn on every swing, which is another important consideration.

Another good practice ball is the Almost Golf Ball, which is a pressurized ball with a semisoft covering that has some of the feel of a real golf ball yet won't fly too far, so you can find it and hit it again. It also won't break windows. There are also yellow foam practice balls that you can find at any major sporting goods retailer. They will work, and even the old reliable Wiffle golf ball versions are serviceable. They don't go far, but if you're slicing, they will slice. But they do not feel like a real golf ball at impact.

There are even indoor practice balls, and in my experience, the best is the Floppy, which is soft enough that you can smack it with a wedge off the sliding glass doors of your living room over and over. The first time I used the Floppy inside, I dropped it on the living room carpet in front of my wife and smacked it with a full swing right off the picture window. My wife nearly fainted until the Floppy smacked the glass with nothing more than a soft thud. We have remained married.

Having good practice golf balls is vital because the golf course and the driving range are not easy learning environments. First of all, there are people watching you, or at least you think they are (actually they probably couldn't care less, but you know what I mean). On the golf course, you can slice fourteen consecutive tee shots and never have the chance to truly assess what's going wrong. Same thing on the range. But at home, you can try things you aren't likely to try elsewhere, like slowing your swing tempo, or experimenting with your backswing path. You can spend an entire evening focusing on one specific goal, like squaring the clubface — always a good idea — without worrying about results. With any of the above-mentioned practice balls, you will get instant feedback.

The next most underrated essential is a good driving range regimen. Or any practice range regimen, because most people don't have one. Most people give more forethought to finding a parking spot at Wal-Mart than to their hour at the range. I know this because I have seen you at the range. Wherever you play, I have seen you.

For example, you always buy the biggest bucket available, right? Is there any swing flaw that a hundred balls can't fix?

You walk past the short-game area and the practice green and think, "I'll finish up there on my way out."

At your hitting station, you grab a 9-iron and launch five or six balls. They don't fly straight, but they are in the air. Good enough.

You reach for the driver. You hit a couple dead straight, then a third. But they don't go as far as you would like. You remember a tip you saw on TV while watching the Masters — something about "firing your left hip." You try that.

The ball rockets off the clubface, 20 yards farther. You keep doing this — it's like magic! Several shots in a row disappear toward the horizon like missiles. You start looking around: Hey, does anybody see how good I'm hitting it over here?

Then one shot goes left. You quickly tee up another. Another ball to the left. You reach for another ball and think about more left hip turn. Oh, no, that's more left. Tee up another. Man, that's left of left. Another ball. You almost hit the guy next to you.

You hastily tee another ball. Wow, that one is way right.

What follows next are the fastest fifty balls you've ever hit. When you finally stop, you are sweating and exasperated. You give up on firing your left hip. You just want to hit it straight again without a thought about the distance. But the ball is going left, then right, and once you almost missed it. Your hands hurt and your back is getting sore. You look down at your bucket; only ten balls left.

Ten balls left to fix my drive! What happened? You take a deep breath and try to relax. You slow your pace and leisurely hit the last ten balls more or less straight, the way you did when you arrived.

You look at your watch. You're late for meeting your spouse. You pack up, passing the practice green in a hustling walk to your car.

"How did the range go?" you are asked later.

"Got my swings in," you say. "It was OK in the end."

Yes, I have seen you before.

In the mirror.

So, why do our practice sessions at the range seem so unproductive?

"Because at the driving range, people hit golf balls," says Laird Small, the 2003 PGA Teacher of the Year and the director of the Pebble Beach Golf Academy. "On the golf course, we have to hit golf shots."

That's more than a cute turn of phrase.

"It would do amateur players a lot of good to attend a pro tournament so they could go to the range and watch the way the pros practice," says Butch Harmon. "The pros never beat balls. They'll hit about twenty-five or thirty balls in an hour. They are simulating real golf where you have to wait between shots.

"Who plays golf by raking one ball after another into the same place while hitting the same club? Nobody, right? So why do people practice like that?"

Every teaching pro I have talked to on this subject said recreational golfers should hit only a small bucket of balls, about thirty minutes' worth, at the range. In that time, they should be working on improving just one thing, whether it's staying in balance or staying in tempo or hitting the ball first rather than the ground. It can be anything, but stick to a small, specific goal.

"You have to have a specific full-swing practice goal, because that practice session goes by very fast," says Mike Bender, listed in the top ten of *Golf Digest*'s teachers nationwide. "It takes about 1.5 seconds to hit a shot. Even if you hit a hundred balls, that's only two and one-half minutes of swinging. So you better have a specific goal if you're going to get something out of two and one-half minutes of practice."

Some golf pros suggest that golfers go to the short-game practice area first to be sure to fit that into their session. At the least, they say, set a time limit for full-swing practice regardless of how things are going.

"People should spend no more than one-third of their time at the range," Bender, who has an academy in Lake Mary, Florida, says. "It could be as high as 50 percent, but only if they just took a lesson and are working on a new swing technique."

The rest of their practice time should be spent on the short game.

Now, I know what you're thinking: Putting and chipping are boring. Seeing good shots soar off your driver is a rush.

"That's part of the love-hate thing in golf," says Bender. "They love to practice their driver. They hate it when they can't break 100. But here's what people have to understand: The full swing is 80 percent technique and 20 percent feel, and the short game is 80 percent feel and 20 percent technique. Improving your short-game feel is much easier and will make your scores drop right away. On the range, people often aren't sure what's going on. Even a bad swing produces good results a few times. Then people try to recapture that moment for the next hour or more. They're spinning their wheels."

Bender and Laird suggested making short-game practice fun by playing games with yourself or a buddy. Try to see, for example, how many 5-foot putts in a row you can make. Have a competition to see who can hit the most chips within 3 feet of the hole. Loser buys the drinks afterward.

Either way you probably save money, because you're buying small practice buckets instead of jumbo ones.

The next most underrated golf essential?

Rain gloves, a rain suit, and waterproof golf shoes. I know that's three things but they're all related. And I know this may sound like I'm now calling for technically elaborate equipment purchases when I've been largely preaching golf minimalism. But the fact is, it does rain out there eventually, and if you're a real golfer, you don't come inside unless there's lightning.

I concede that I used to all but give up at the sight of a decent downpour, and I know a lot of people who still do. The Scots have a saying: "Nae wind, nae rain, nae golf." In much of America, it's more like "Rain? Wind? And the cart girl went in? I'm outta here."

But I've come to see that successfully playing in the rain is a mindset. It is not hard, or terribly expensive, to be prepared for rain, and you get to play more that way. As with most things in modern golf, new equipment can also help considerably. These days, we have it pretty good in sloppy conditions. For the best advice on playing well in the rain, I scoured the list of *Golf Magazine*'s top one hundred teachers for someone with a deep background in getting wet on the links. I came upon Jerry Mowlds, who grew up in Oregon, turned professional four decades ago, and is the director of instruction at the spectacular Pumpkin Ridge Golf Club outside Portland.

Mowlds told me all his tricks, like how he stores a few old regular gloves in a plastic bag inside his golf bag. "That can get you through eighteen holes easily," he said. But sometimes it's raining too hard for a regular glove. So he always has rain gloves, which are made with a fabric that grips better when wet. They cost about $20. "I am sure every tour pro has rain gloves in the bag," Mowlds said.

Mowlds also said to buy a waterproof rain suit made for golf, or at least for athletics, not one for duck hunting or watching a holiday parade in a mist. This is the biggest expense ($200 to $800), but you should get one, or at least an inexpensive one. Why? Consider how many days there will be in the next three golf seasons when rain may ruin a golf round you were looking forward to playing. If it's more than one a year, given the price of greens fees, the suit will probably pay for itself in four years. The majority of golfers won't fork over the expense of a rain suit. I know I went through a stage when I tried to get by with a heavy windbreaker and lots of towels whenever it rained. That was a mistake. But we make bizarre choices. We think nothing of spending $100 to play golf for one day but won't spend $400 on a quality rain suit that might last ten years and allow us to enjoy forty more golf rounds when it's raining. So think of it as an extra $10 for every round it rains. You spend that on a hot dog and drink at the turn.

A good rain suit should have a few components. First of all, it shouldn't make all kinds of swishy sounds when you swing or walk. New stretchy materials eliminate all that noise. Since it will probably be slipped on over your regular golf outfit, the rain suit should have two-way or sturdy, wide zippers. Most of the jackets have a high storm collar to keep the rain off your neck and back. One company, Zero Restriction, makes several good models. So does Columbia.

Waterproof shoes, meanwhile, are everywhere in the golf market-place now, and there's no reason not to have one pair. "Playing in the rain used to be a mess; people don't realize how good they have it now," Mowlds said. "Our shoes, socks, and feet would be soaked by the time we got to the first green. Nowadays, with all the waterproof shoes, everybody is dry. But people buy a $70 pair of cheaper golf shoes instead of paying another $70 for something waterproof. Even if it's not raining the day you play, it might have rained the day before. Do you want to step in a soft puddle on the first hole and have a waterlogged sock and shoe for the next four hours? Just spend the extra money."

Speaking of money, the last of my most underrated golf essentials is the cheapest by far. It is the banana. It comes in its own easy-opening wrapper. It travels extremely well, including in a golf bag unless you forget it is there. Its yellow color matches well with the green — or brown — of every golf course. Golfers worry about how to replenish themselves on the golf course and spend way too much money on pre-wrapped sandwiches and expensive energy bars. A simple banana has fiber and ample quantities of vitamins B and C and loads of potassium, which helps restock electrolytes. That's why you see so many tour pros eating bananas on the course. It's an easy, quick refueling stop.

Underrated? You bet. A ripe banana in the bag might be worth a stroke per nine holes. One other thing a banana won't do — it won't stain your shirt, pants, or skirt if you accidentally drop it. That can't be said for a hot dog with mustard. And that's no myth.

Debunking myths and falsehoods is fun. It will make golf essentially easier. But remember, this is still golf. No other sport will test you in the same way. Sam Snead and Ted Williams were once discussing what was harder, hitting a golf ball or a baseball. Snead acknowledged the golf ball wasn't moving but added: "You don't have to go up in the stands and play your foul balls. I do."

Think about that for a while. If it helps, remember, we're never alone. Golf mistreats us equally in the end. It also lifts us up. The ultimate essential remains the understanding that this odd, unique game we play demands a singular skill at finding the silver lining and moving forward to the next shot. This coming from a golfer who wrapped a pitching wedge around a tree while just practicing. But distorting golf's often brutal reality is a golf essential.

I am certain that during one of the earliest golf matches in the fifteenth century along the Firth of Forth in eastern Scotland, a beleaguered sheepherder missed a 3-foot putt when his rounded stone lipped out of a rabbit hole. He considered flinging his stick in the direction of the North Sea but instead reminded himself that he was getting better at this new game, he would improve if he just practiced a little more diligently, and besides, that rabbit hole was irregular and too small for such a good putt anyway.

Then, as the other sheepherders trudged away, he slammed his stick into the little bag he was carrying on his shoulder. He felt better.

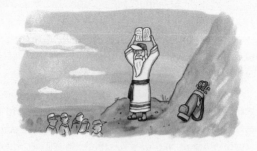

2

The Rules of Golf

If you think it's hard to meet new people,
try picking up the wrong golf ball.

JACK LEMMON

THERE ARE ALL kinds of hazards, little hidden tricks, and deceptions in the game of golf that go unheeded by unsuspecting golfers. We golfers tend to dress nicely, smile at the appropriate times, and mind our manners, so naturally we expect fairness and decency from golf in return. Ha, we are fools. This is golf. Golf flouts righteousness. Here are just a few examples:

Many tee boxes do not point toward the fairway, so many tee shots do not go there either. Everyone thinks these are routine errant shots, when in fact we probably have just been duped, too naive to think the golf course itself is conspiring against us. Most people have the wrong loft on their putter — you probably didn't even know a putter had loft. But your trusty putter may be working against you. Golf suspends simple math skills. In other words, people cheat. The sand in bunkers, as organic and untreated a material as there is, is rarely evenhanded. The sand can be thicker and heavier in some bunkers than it is in other bunkers, so what was a beautiful par-saving swing in a bunker on the first hole becomes a triple-bogey disaster swing in the bunker on the fourth hole. Even the sand in different parts of the *same* bunker can vary. Meanwhile, a small army of scientists and engineers — holed away in an unnoticed New Jersey bunker (not the sand kind) — actually govern golf. And don't you dare cross them.

But more than anything else, lording over all pertinent things in golf, there is the Rules of Golf, the most complex, shadowy, and abstruse document known to this world or probably any other. In fact, if big-brained aliens ever land on Earth and ask for a book that explains how we administer society, we ought to hand them the 138-page Rules of Golf because it would so consume and distract them we would have plenty of time to steal all their technological secrets and make off with their futuristic weapons. The Rules of Golf can overpower any brain.

Notice, of course, that I capitalized the *R* in *Rules*, because that's what officious, I mean official, Rules gurus always do. This is true. Why? Because the golf rule book refers to the rules as Rules, and the highly serious people who shepherd the Rules at the United States Golf Association — and someone must — do everything exactly as the rule book states.

For example, those are not sand traps on your local golf course. They are most decidedly bunkers. It's not a pin propped in the hole on the first green, it's a flagstick. It is not the tee box but the teeing ground. This is true because these are three of fifty defined terms in the Rules of Golf, and they are always used by Rules officials and never substituted with other inappropriate slang golf terms.

Once I got an inebriated Rules official to utter the words *sand trap* and *tee box*, by bribing him with a free beer. The next morning he shamefully turned in his Rules badge. Actually, that's not true. Well, the second part of the story isn't true.

Some other common golf terms that are not in the Rules even if they are part of the universal vernacular of America's 28 million golfers:

Puddle: Don't be silly. That little collection of rain where your ball ended up is "casual water." You often get relief from casual water. Snow or natural ice, incidentally, can also be called casual water. But manufactured ice is an "obstruction" (different Rule). That's right, if Mother Nature has made the ice your ball ends up in, you're in good shape, but if you hit your ball into your mother's paper cup of Scotch on the rocks, which is, of course, just down to the ice, you're checking into a completely different Rule and resolution (not to mention having to buy Mom another drink).

And don't embarrass yourself trying to call dew and frost on the golf course casual water. No Rule. No relief. Don't even go there.

Dirt: If it has a line drawn around it, it is "ground under repair" (that's good for you because you can probably move the ball). No line? Sorry, bad news. Don't bother looking around beseechingly at your golfing partners when this happens. We know you got jobbed. But what can we do? It's the Rules with a capital *R*.

Cup: It's a "hole" and the white thing inside it is the "lining." I have no idea how many beers it would take to get a Rules official to use the word *cup*, but it would be so many you probably wouldn't be able to understand what was said anyway.

Snake: As in "My ball came to rest on a dead snake so I'm not hitting it." Actually, the snake, if dead, is an "outside agency" and you must play the ball off it. If the snake were alive, you could drop another ball safely away from the snake.

Bad luck. Stupid game. Really unfair: All common terms that might be spoken — or screamed — if your ball was bouncing down the center of the fairway until it hit a rock, or a squirrel, and deflected into the woods. This is upsetting because that's where you must play your next stroke from. The Rules have a definition for this outcome. It's officially recognized as the "rub of the green."

In other words: Stop your whining. Besides, your casual water tears are messing up the teeing ground as I aim at the flagstick above the hole several feet from a bunker.

Anyway, when it comes to the Rules, I have found that all golfers are separated into three categories:

1. The happy clueless. These are golfers who know almost no Rules and have no interest in learning them. These are also known as tennis players, fraternity brothers using golf as an excuse to get drunk, and people at a convention playing their one round of golf a year.

2. The happy and mostly uneducated. These are golfers who know some Rules but not all of them, and they think trying to learn all of them is pointless because the Rules are too convoluted. They have learned some simple edicts and now want to be left alone. These golfers make up 85 percent of the golfing public.

3. The happy prosecutors. These are golfers who know all the Rules and almost all of the hundreds of decisions handed down over hundreds of years to penalize and persecute the rest of us. These people are known as golf Rules Nazis. They are as popular as most Nazis.

The truth is there is no hope for categories 1 and 3 but much hope for those in the middle. For the happy and mostly uneducated, there are about ten basic, relatively easy rules that everyone should know and understand. They are also the most abused. So:

Ten Essential Rules to Remember (with Painless Translations)

Be One with Your Ball

Before you start your round, you must be able to identify the ball you are playing. When two or three people hit into the same cluster of trees off the first tee, you are not supposed to say, "I think I hit a Top-Flite, or a Titleist, or a Tour-something. It definitely began with a *T*."

This is not nitpicking, especially for beginners who spray the ball just a bit. If you don't know what ball you hit, trust me, it will happen that you and one of your playing partners will drive a ball from the tee into roughly the same place, and when you get there neither of you will know what ball you played. Or, if you both know the brand but not the number of the ball you played, it is an unlucky certainty that you'll find both balls — same brand, probably Titleist — but you will never know whose ball is whose because you don't know the number.

(By the way — not that I advise doing this on a crowded muni on a Sunday afternoon — but by the Rules, both of you would have to declare your ball lost and return to the tee to hit what would now be your third shot.)

So at the least, know what brand of ball you're playing and the number. If you want to be safer, mark your ball with a pen or a Sharpie to identify it. Avoid drawing a smiley face; it tends to mock you from a terrible lie in the rough.

Bag Check

If you want to carry sixteen clubs in your bag because you're trying out two putters and an extra driver, at least know that you are violating the Rule that permits just fourteen clubs. You probably mean no harm, and there's always room for experimenting, but your playing partners may want to get a little side bet going, and they could have an opinion about your extra baggage.

You may see this as ridiculous — you can't hit the fourteen clubs you already have straight so why would two more uncooperative clubs matter? But other golfers will perceive it as an advantage because they, in their own golfer delusional way, might like to carry sixteen clubs, believing that today is the day they will successfully hit a 2-iron.

So remember, fourteen clubs is the limit. As simple as that is, guys get penalized on the pro tours for this all the time. In 2001 at the British Open, the diminutive Welshman Ian Woosnam was near the lead heading into the final round when his caddie forgot to take out an extra driver Woosnam had been experimenting with on the practice range. When Woosnam discovered he had fifteen clubs on the second tee, he called the two-stroke penalty on himself. Woosnam's nickname is "Wee Woozy," and boy, was he ever on that second tee.

While he finished three strokes behind the winner, the tournament might have had a different outcome had Wee Woozy been two strokes closer throughout the final round, putting pressure on the leader.

This is a good Rule, an elementary way to make sure everyone has the same tools, although it is a truth that most of us would probably do better with ten clubs. Less thinking that way.

Teeing Off

You can tee your ball at or just behind the imaginary line drawn between the front of the tee markers, but you don't have to. This, in fact, is usually where you'll find the most divots and inadequate grass. You can tee your ball up to two club lengths back from the markers, while staying between them. You won't miss the extra 3 feet, but you might get a flatter, smoother lie.

Tee boxes, excuse me, the teeing ground, is notoriously bumpy and uneven, especially in certain climates and at municipal courses where the budget probably isn't big enough to pay for frequent rolling of the tees. There is level ground, but you should look for it instead of just sticking a tee in the middle of the markers. More important: Make sure your feet will be level, and level with the ball. Many a slice occurs because the ball is subtly below your feet, even if it's only half an inch.

As for the tee markers pointing you the wrong way, make sure you don't fall for this trick. Golf architects design their layouts to protect par. Often the design of the entire hole is to lure the golfer to hit it right on a dogleg left or toward a particularly punitive bunker complex. To maximize the number of balls rolling or flying in that direction, the architect might build the tee box so that the long sides of its rectangular shape create an alley that points directly toward the trouble. This is exceedingly common and exceedingly overlooked.

Don't use the markers to take aim! They are not there to help you. And here's another reason to ignore those markers: At many golf courses, the tee markers might be moved every other day so that the grass can be mowed.

Who do you think puts those tee markers back in place after the mowing? At some very select courses it might be a maintenance worker trained to look where he's jabbing the tee markers in the ground so that they are aligned to create an aiming corridor pointing toward the fairway or green. At most courses, it's just somebody who at five thirty in the morning couldn't care less where your shot ends up. He's just in a hurry to get eighteen tee boxes mowed by six thirty.

Out-of-Bounds Options

If you hit your ball out-of-bounds, you must hit another ball from the same spot as the original shot, or as near to it as possible. If on the tee, you can re-tee. Out-of-bounds areas are defined by white stakes. There is a one-stroke penalty. If you're not sure if your shot went out, announce that you are hitting a provisional ball. You must declare it. If you find the original shot in bounds, great. If not, play the provisional.

The out-of-bounds Rule may be the most controversial commonly applied Rule in golf. Many people think it should be changed because it slows play, puts pressure on people to go back to the tee, and is overly punitive. As TV golf commentator and teacher Peter Kostis points out, you are penalized less for whiffing the ball on the tee (one-stroke penalty but at least you're hitting two) than you are for hitting it off the tee and out of play (back to the tee and hitting three or you hit a provisional and you still lie three). Kostis and others suggest that out-of-bounds areas should be treated like lateral water hazards (more on that Rule later). But essentially, if you hit it out-of-bounds, you would instead drop two club lengths from the point where the ball went out-of-bounds with a one-stroke penalty. You would still be hitting three, but you've gained the distance of your errant shot.

Many recreational golfers already play out-of-bounds shots this way. And if you and your friends want to substitute your own interpretation of the lost-ball Rule for a day, week, year, or lifetime, that's perfectly fine. Just know what the Rule actually is. Because you won't be playing every round with your friends or you might end up in a friendly, or not friendly, competition. Remember, Rules Nazis are lurking out there.

The safest way to proceed in these conditions? Hit a provisional unless you positively see the ball.

I'm just trying to protect you. It may not be the fairest Rule, but it is an easy one to understand and recall.

Lose a Ball? See "Out-of-Bounds"

If you hit a ball and think it's lost, the Rule is the same as for a ball hit out-of-bounds. If you didn't see where it went or if it looked as if it was heading for the cemetery across the highway, accept the likely mortality of your shot. Hit a provisional. You are allowed five minutes to look for the first ball.

This is another controversial and oft-ignored Rule, sometimes with good reason. You can leave the tee all but certain your tee shot is just over a hump in the right rough. It's so obvious where it is that you don't hit a provisional. Everyone in your group saw where it went and assured you it should be OK. But unbeknownst to your group, wild fescue is growing just beyond the hump. Again, if playing a competition or in a league, you must head back to the tee. If it's a hot day, likely the pace of play is really slow, and even more likely, there's another group waiting on the tee. At that point I'm not sure it's even safe to go back to the tee and whack another one. So there will be a lot of pressure to just drop a ball and take a stroke.

This has led some people to lobby that this Rule be changed just like the out-of-bounds Rule. The problem is that unlike the out-of-bounds situation, where you probably saw the OB ahead of time and probably saw the ball fly or roll toward that area so you can estimate its general location, a lost ball can occur in a multitude of ways, some completely unexplainable.

Lost balls are just that: lost. In many cases, no one saw where the ball went so no one can accurately say where it was last seen or where it should be placed. What if no one ever saw it off the club? Or lost the ball in the sun or a cloud? Where do you drop the ball then?

Losing your ball definitely costs you strokes. One of the most fundamental tenets of playing golf: Try not to lose your ball.

And, of course, hit a provisional if you have any doubt where it is.

Divining Water Hazards

If you hit a ball into a water hazard, typically defined by yellow stakes, you can always try playing it out of the hazard, which could work if you don't mind playing the rest of the day with mud in your hair. Otherwise, you have two options: the now-familiar play-it-from-the-spot-of-the-previous-shot option, or — and pay attention, because this is the most misunderstood Rule in golf — you can drop a ball behind the water hazard. But you must keep the point where the original ball last crossed the margin of the hazard between you and the hole.

What does that mean? Look at the flagstick and draw an imaginary line from it to the point where your ball last crossed the margin of the hazard. Now visualize that line going backward for hundreds of yards. You can drop your ball anywhere on that line. Be imaginative where you drop on the line because sometimes going back 100 yards is to your advantage. Sometimes going back 40 feet gives you a flatter surface to hit from.

This happens at the Masters on the par-5 fifteenth hole every year. A steep hill precedes the pond in front of the green, and it is a much more precipitous slope than the television cameras reveal. Golfers who dunk their balls in that pond tend to go back anywhere from 50 to 100 yards, both to set up a familiar shot and to get some reasonably level ground.

So don't let the frustration of plunking your ball in the water lead you to another mistake. And don't just go up and drop a ball a few feet behind the water. That's not the Rule — find the appropriate line. Now in some cases, usually par 3s, a clearly marked drop area is identified or circled in white paint. This is usually your best choice if there is one.

And if you walk around the pond or hazard and drop on the other side of the water — the side closer to the green — you must believe in the tooth fairy. I do see people do this all the time and I wonder: Under what circumstances would a game as difficult as golf give you a free pass like that? Of course, the Rules are most likely going to make you hit it over the water again.

More Water, with a Twist

If you hit a ball into a lateral water hazard, which is a pond, lake, swamp, or ocean where it is deemed impractical to drop behind the hazard, you have all the same options. You will know it is a lateral water hazard if it is defined by red stakes. As mentioned earlier, the Rules also allow players to choose one of two other options. The one used most frequently, after taking a one-stroke penalty, is dropping the ball within two club lengths of the point where it last crossed the margin of the hazard, no nearer the hole. You can also drop a ball on a point on the opposite margin of the water hazard equidistant from the hole.

Accept the Hand You Are Dealt

All right, enough of the water hazards. It's depressing just talking about them. Here is a Rule so elementary, so clear and easily understood, so unambiguous, and so easy to comply with that you would think it would never be broken except by accident. Yet, it might be the most broken Rule of all — and not often by accident.

It's the ball "played as it lies" Rule. It is Rule 13, just to make it sound more ominous. So that means don't roll the ball over to better grass. Don't jostle it with your club to get it sitting up on top of the grass instead of buried in it. You can't improve your lie or stance at all — ever.

You can't do what my cousin Jerry used to do.

Me: "Got a good lie over there, Jerry?"

Jerry (as he repeatedly pressed his club head behind his ball in the rough): "Not yet."

It is best to get used to the concept that golf is basically a game in which you hit the ball, find it, and hit it again. There are exceptions, but it means reading the rule book carefully. Few exceptions deal with shots in plain view resting in the fairway or rough.

Once you get used to playing the ball as it lies, you will rarely think about it, even if you get a bad break. Others will respect you for it. There does seem to be a good karma that envelops those who embrace this approach to the game. If you take your medicine, things will be fine. Like, for example, those odd instances when your ball comes to rest in an old divot. Maybe it's because I'm concentrating more on hitting the ball first — not a bad idea — but those shots always seem to turn out OK. Not necessarily perfect but not worth getting your shorts in an angry knot about, which really hurts your hip turn anyway.

Thinking of Clearing a Path? Don't Bust That Stupid Twig

All of us at one time or another get into a position in which the removal of one little tree limb or sprig of a bush would give us a clear shot at the green. Guess what? You cannot break off that twig or bend that sprig. You cannot even break it by accident with a practice swing. Nice try, though.

This may also seem unfair. Why be penalized for breaking a twig if it was an accident? Because the Rules cannot be sure it was by accident. Two or three hearty, aggressive practice swings, with the club cutting the brush like a scythe, can turn a deadly lie in tall grass to an agreeable one. If your opponent did that, you would want the Rules to prevent it.

Leave the Counseling to Caddies

This is the last, and largely unknown, Rule that everyone should know. It is against the Rules to give advice on the golf course, unless you are a caddie or a partner in a match. That means you are allowed to tell that know-it-all in your group to stop breaking the Rules with all the swing tips, sand shot advice, and putting grip instruction.

See, and you thought the Rules only penalized you. They can be on your side after all.

Now, as much as I've been making fun of Rules officials, all golfers should know they are very real people. It's likely that some of them probably even wait in line next to you at the grocery store, and you are completely unaware!

All golfers should understand how helpful the men and women watching over our golf Rules can be, not just to officiate your local tournament or club championship, but to settle arguments. While it is true that many golfers have a sketchy understanding of the Rules, it does not stop most of them from getting into Rules arguments on a daily basis all over the country. In prime golf season, I get five e-mails a week from readers wanting me to settle Rules situations that arose recently in their group.

That is always good fun. Since I am not an actual Rules official, I tell them whatever comes into my mind that day. I've tried telling them that the penalty for hitting it out-of-bounds is to hop on one foot while patting the top of your head and singing "Dixie."

I don't know if anyone out there has actually believed me. But if someday while playing golf you hear someone warbling "Dixie" while hopping on one foot, you will know that person reads *The New York Times.*

But back to the real Rules officials. On any given weekend in America, there might be a Rules argument for every birdie made. Wait a minute; the average score of the average golfer is still 100. Obviously, there are way more arguments than birdies.

When these arguments reach a certain fevered pitch, someone usually asks an elder on the scene whom everyone recognizes as somewhat of a Rules guru. But that elder is going to render an opinion that contradicts one side of the argument, and that will leave someone still feeling wronged. If that party is sufficiently aggrieved — or nineteenth-hole lubricated — then a call or e-mail will be placed to the United States Golf Association headquarters in Far Hills, New Jersey.

People call the USGA because since 1894, the organization has governed a national championship, and shortly thereafter it devised, interpreted, and oversaw the Rules of Golf as played in the United States. The first golf rules, or the first written golf rules, were jotted down by the Gentlemen Golfers of Leith of Scotland in 1744. (This group is now called the Honourable Company of Edinburgh Golfers.) There were essentially thirteen rules, establishing things like what to do if your ball lands in water or is lost (pretty much the same rules as now). Believe it or not, the Gentlemen Golfers of Leith also addressed what to do if your ball strikes a horse or a dog. It must be "played as it lyes." The rule persists, if not the Old English spelling.

In 1897, the Royal and Ancient Golf Club (R&A) of St. Andrews, Scotland, took over the role of watching over golf's rules east of the Atlantic Ocean. For decades, the Rules of Golf were slightly different on each side of the Atlantic. The ball size was different, for example, and at various times you could use a steel-shafted club in the United States but not in Britain. The same was true when it came to a center-shafted putter or certain kinds of wedges. In 1952, the USGA and the R&A came to agreement on almost all the Rules (the ball size remained different for nearly another three decades). These Rules are now officially recognized for almost all competitive play. And so, more than one hundred years after the founding of the USGA, when average American golfers are stumped by something about the Rules or how to apply them, they phone up the USGA.

And these phone calls are not a random occurrence. Rules officials at the USGA answer 20,000 Rules queries every year. The USGA offices are not open on weekends, but late on Sunday afternoons, especially during the summer, the telephone at the main switchboard rings nonetheless.

"It will be three guys on a speakerphone from the nineteenth hole at some club," according to Genger Fahleson, the USGA director of Rules education. "They have a golf Rules question and they want an answer."

The security guard who answers these calls is trained to ascertain if the outcome of a live tournament or club championship is at stake. Questions that can wait a day will be directed to a USGA Rules associate's voice mail. "But if there is some bona fide competitive event involved, the guard has cell phone numbers for the Rules officials," Fahleson said. "He will get in touch with us, and we will call back and make a ruling."

So somewhere at one of the roughly 16,000 golf courses in America, some golfer who did or did not mark a ball properly or did or did not move a bunker rake improperly will be penalized or exonerated. A scorecard will be accepted or adjusted. Another golf day in America will end with a specific tally of a specific number of strokes — all thanks to a USGA Rules official who probably stepped away from a Sunday barbecue to offer an expert decision. If this sounds unusual, or excessive, then you have no grasp of just how obsessed golfers can be with the Rules of Golf, or how necessary they are in managing the game. And you certainly haven't sat at the desk of a USGA Rules associate.

Monday through Friday, forty hours a week, it is the full-time job of a Rules associate to answer the phone calls, e-mail messages, and mailings of everyday golfers who are perplexed or confounded by some element of the Rules. "They come in year-round but we are busiest from late May to September," Fahleson said. "When we leave on a Friday, it's not unusual for the Rules e-mail in box to be empty. When we come back Monday morning, there are several hundred questions in there." In most other sports, be it beer-league softball or youth soccer, there is an umpire, referee, or official presiding over the action to make decisions and enforce rulings. In golf, 99 percent of the time, the players are on their own, trying to figure out what the appropriate ruling should be. And clearly, many people have never seen a golf rule book. Most people have never read it, and those who have aren't likely to have committed it to memory.

"We do try to make the Rules as simple as possible, but we're dealing with a game played across thousands of acres, with so many outside factors like weather and wildlife," said Bernie Loehr, USGA manager for the Rules of Golf. "There are a lot of situations that can happen and so many possibilities to consider."

For example, because I love questions about golf and animals, what if a golf ball hit near but not in a water hazard lodges beneath the shell of a turtle, and the turtle then dives into the water hazard with the ball? (You are allowed to drop a ball as near as possible to where the turtle was when the ball struck it, no penalty.) What if the ball got lodged in the turtle's shell while the turtle was floating in the pond? (Proceed as if you hit your ball into a hazard, one penalty stroke.) What if the ball lodges in the turtle's shell outside the pond, but the turtle is dead? (We know this answer: You may either play it as it lies without penalty or declare your ball unplayable, taking one penalty stroke.)

Most of the questions forwarded to the USGA receive a response in ten to fifteen business days, which takes some doing when the queries are arriving by the thousands. There are two full-time Rules associates, in addition to Loehr, Fahleson, and nine regional directors who may answer up to forty questions a month. Other USGA staff members occasionally pitch in to help as well.

And yes, while most questions take the Rules associates just thirty seconds to answer, some Rules situations can temporarily stump the USGA officials. In that case, the Rules gurus gather in the office hall. The group may take a vote on what the ruling is. And if something similar comes up again and again, the officials may ask the Rules of Golf Committee to make a decision. "That's the fascinating thing about the Rules of Golf," Fahleson said. "They're kind of like the game of golf. You can never completely master it."

I wondered if at social gatherings or parties, being a Rules official is like being a doctor — everyone has a question. "People will invariably say, 'I got one for you,'" said Loehr, who joined the USGA when he retired as a comptroller in 2004. "And they give you a Rules situation. It's OK; I like the Rules."

What's the most common question? You guessed it: lost-ball or out-of-bounds queries. And the staff at the USGA, like me, is astounded by the number of people who think they can drop their ball on the green side of a hazard when the ball they hit did not carry the hazard. Then there are the knuckleheads — I can call them that because I think I'm part of the group — who wonder about crazy, wacky possibilities. You know, what if my drive collides with a low-flying aircraft? Or what if everyone sees my ball roll into the hole, but when we get there, we can't find it?

"When the conversation begins with 'what if,' we know that what follows may not be reasonable," Loehr said. "Sometimes you have to ask, 'Guys, did this really happen?'"

To help educate the golfing public, the USGA Web site (www.usga .org) has a vast listing of frequently asked questions pertaining to each of the thirty-four primary Rules. There are Rules videos and quizzes as well, because the USGA wants golfers to embrace the Rules, not be puzzled by them. But in the end, when there's a difference of opinion about golf procedure or about which Rule applies to a thorny situation, the phone will ring at the grand USGA headquarters. "Sometimes you'll give them the ruling, and over the speakerphone you'll hear people cheering in the background," Loehr said. "Someone will say, 'Thanks, Bernie, we owe you a beer.'

"I've never collected, but I'm probably owed a lot of beers all over the country."

Why We Cheat (and Guess Who's Watching)

There is another reason the Rules exist. It's to identify when someone is cheating, although many times I don't think we need a rule book to do that. But this is another unseen part of the game. How unseen?

In a recent online poll of more than 7,000 golfers, 70 percent said they cheated on the course. Ninety-five percent said they were not caught, or at least no one said anything. A 2002 survey of 400 top business executives reported that 82 percent admitted to cheating at golf. Around the same time, PGA Tour caddies were questioned about cheating, and 26 percent said they had seen players cheat on tour.

Wow. What a bunch of cheaters!

Well, let's be real. On the recreational level, some of this is probably the mathematics ruse that people like to pull occasionally. What did Will Rogers say? "Income tax has made liars out of more people than golf has."

So just as they might with their taxes, people can get a little forgetful. I don't know if it's the smell of freshly cut grass or the proximity to pond water, but something about the golf course disrupts people's grade-school arithmetic. Calculating the number of strokes taken on a hole, which would be easy work for a six-year-old, becomes vexing to golfers. Maybe it's the golf cart fumes. But after many a tough hole, an 8 or a 7 gets marked down as a 6. There are much more inventive ways to cheat on the golf course; some of them are mildly amusing. There's the old reliable foot wedge (your toe moves a ball a few feet to a better lie). There's the bait-and-switch (hit a rock-hard distance ball off the tee, then switch to a soft premium ball to putt with on the green). Some people seem to magically "find" wayward balls that were presumed lost by all who saw the shot. I have heard of golfers who rip holes in their pockets so they can surreptitiously drop a ball through the pant leg onto the ground.

Voilà! "Here it is. I found it!"

It's possible people do these things because they come to golf with experience playing other sports, where cheating is all but sanctioned on some level. In soccer or ice hockey, players pretend to be fouled to influence a referee's call. Baseball catchers try to pull wayward pitches back toward the strike zone, hoping to get a strike call from the umpire. Basketball players are taught to use their bodies to shield opponents from the ball in ways that skirt the rules or blur them. Football linemen hold on almost every play. The list of ways that subtle, or overt, cheating takes place in sport is lengthy. These acts are placed in a gray area, something essentially not illegal.

In golf, such a gray area would exist only in a player's conscience because unlike in nearly all other sports, the players call the violations on themselves. The standards set are very high. Not only can a player in a tournament be disqualified for cheating; his or her opponent can also be disqualified for witnessing it and not reporting it.

But many golfers, probably not an insignificant number, find bending the Rules totally harmless. It's another unseen part of the game.

I've had scores of people tell me that what they are doing is not cheating because they don't keep score anyway. Other people tell me they break a few Rules because they play so infrequently it's no fun if they don't help themselves occasionally. And I can see their point. I personally can think back to times as a younger player when a form of temporary insanity came over me on the golf course. An outcome on a given hole would seem so unfair and implausible — ever hit the flagstick on the fly and had the ball ricochet into a water hazard? — that I would refuse to write down my real score on my scorecard. Is that cheating? Well, it certainly wasn't truthful, and as I got older I realized no golf hole was worth feeling dishonest.

But there is another realm of golf cheating that deals with the things people do to win matches or to be able to say they had the low score in that day's foursome — or worse, to win a club championship. People do a lot of not-so-harmless things in pursuit of those goals.

"Because golf is a game where an individual score is assigned to every player, there is intense pressure to be good at it, or at least not bad at it," said Dr. Wayne Glad, an Illinois clinical psychologist who has worked extensively with college and pro athletes, including golfers. "In a business setting, people believe they won't nail down the big deal if they are a really terrible player out on the golf course. Plus, there's the sense that everyone else is pretty good, which isn't actually true. But people feel that way. People want to save face."

Dr. Glad added: "Then there are the people who are just incredibly competitive. They feel like they should do whatever it takes to win."

This extends to the pro golf tours, even though in the golf community, there is no more damaging aspersion than to be labeled a cheat. Dr. Glad said that the PGA Tour players he tutors are aware of colleagues who cheat, albeit in devious ways. "They'll talk to each other about certain guys," Glad said. "They'll say, 'You ever notice how often so-and-so coughs in your backswing?'"

On the recreational level, some of the cheating is inadvertent because of a naiveté about the Rules. But I do believe another factor driving people to cheat is the sense that everyone else is doing it. However, there is a big difference between taking a 7 instead of an 8 on a hole that you lost to your opponent anyway and kicking a ball out from under a tree during an important match when you think no one is looking.

And I have witnessed that too often. It is a sick feeling to witness someone you know cheating like that. It is even worse when the person turns and realizes you were watching. Now, I don't care what you think about how hard or how unfair golf is; that is cheating.

It's like what your mother or father told you: You know in your heart when something you are about to do is wrong. And most of us truly believe if you push the golf gods far enough, if you wash yourself in that kind of bad karma, eventually the golf gods will punish you. Maybe somebody somewhere has cheated golf and won in the end. But I doubt it.

Cheating at golf is not always performed by the individual golfer. Sometimes it is institutional or systematic. Go to the back of any large golf magazine and you will come across advertisements for golf balls that fly 25 yards farther than normal golf balls. There are grip alignment aids and devices you can attach to your putter head to hit more putts straight.

Many of these devices work, but according to the Rules, if you use them you are cheating. In the opinion of most golfers, they're illegal, too. It is the same thing with the PGA and LPGA pros. It is a little-known fact that the pro golf tours are not compelled to go by the Rules of Golf; they simply choose to. Golf's rule book devotes dozens of pages to equipment, including incredibly specific dictums on tees, balls, clubs, grips, and everything else in your bag. The angle at which the club shaft connects to the club head is regulated; so are the dimension of the club head and, of course, the grooves on the clubface. These rules also evolve. For instance, the accepted depth and shape of the grooves for irons were changed — after much debate — in 2010.

So yes, people make tees, balls, and clubs that will do amazing things. They're just not within the Rules. At the same time, it is the job of club and ball makers everywhere to design their products so that they are at the very limit of legal guidelines without overstepping them. Still, the temptation to go just a bit farther is always there. Fortunately, someone is monitoring every product made with an amazing conscientiousness that could happen only in golf.

Inside a low-slung building off a nondescript road in a quiet central New Jersey suburb is the most powerful room in golf. It is the orderly laboratory of the USGA Research and Test Center. In this modest building surrounded by rolling, grassy fields, a staff of eighteen decrees which clubs, balls, grips, tees, and devices conform to the Rules.

The designs for new balls, clubs, and golf devices pour into the USGA laboratory by the thousands each year. Getting a stamp of conformity from within those walls could be the difference between a great idea left to languish in a garage and a groundbreaking club that finds its niche in golf's $40 billion industry.

A majority of submissions to the USGA come from golf industry giants like TaylorMade, Titleist, Nike, Callaway, and Ping, but as much as 25 percent are sent to the test center from individuals unaffiliated with any company. Their submissions run the gamut — three-headed putters, balls laced with gunpowder, or gloves with padding promoting a certain grip. Each of those ideas was classified as nonconforming. There are, however, just as many ideas, if not more, that have been accepted. Last year, more than 60 percent of submissions were approved.

You might wonder why the USGA doesn't give its approval to a tee that prevents a slice. Wouldn't that just make the game better and more fun?

"It's about making the skill of the golfer the most important thing, not the golfer's equipment," said John Spitzer, the center's assistant technical director. "It might seem crazy, but if we didn't draw some lines, it could get out of control pretty easily. It's pretty easy to manipulate a club to hit the ball straight, and you could easily make a ball that goes 320 yards even with an average swing. So yes, it's about hitting a little ball, but without the challenge, it's not a game, either."

It would be like cheating. The big manufacturers continue to push the envelope with products that do make a considerable difference. The modern golf balls do go significantly farther than ones made even ten years ago. New clubs are perimeter-weighted so fewer shots fly sideways. The new wave of drivers, made with lighter shafts that generate greater club head speed, routinely outpace older models by 20 to 30 yards. Putters are balanced with space-age materials rather than raw metals. Putters now have variable loft, too, which is more important than you may realize. It's a little-known fact that a golf ball at rest on a green actually sits in a tiny indentation in the grass caused by the weight of the ball. A putter may be nicknamed the flat stick, but like a lot of nicknames, that is not very accurate. A putter typically has loft in the range of 3 to 5 degrees. The loft helps lift the ball out of the indentation and get it rolling. Depending on your putting style, you might need more or less loft. The result: truer putts thanks to technology (sadly, we still tend to aim wrong).

The hundreds of engineers employed by major manufacturers know all these things and know how to capitalize on them. They come up with literally hundreds of new ideas every year, some that in the eyes of the USGA go too far.

"The big companies are trying to help their customers play better," Spitzer said. "We understand that and have allowed much progress. So we are not trying to preserve the game, but we are trying to protect it."

Protecting the game means putting every proposed new club through a mad scientist's catalog of lab tests. The shaft is bent, the head measured, and the grip analyzed. There's a shadowgraph test and another test for checking the club's moment of inertia. The club's volume is checked and its surface roughness gauged. Spin rates off the face are calculated — and not just in normal conditions; another test uses synthetic fabric to mimic wet grass. Golf balls, if possible, seem to face additional scrutiny. They are weighed, measured, sometimes sliced open or compressed. Most are shot by a mini cannon through a 75-foot tunnel past infrared sensors and lasers with dozens of readouts produced. Other balls are hit by a mechanical golfer across a long driving range where trajectory monitors designed to follow missiles aimed at warships instead wait in the grass to chart the path of each ball. Even after a ball is deemed to be conforming, the USGA sleuths are not done. They will visit a local Dick's Sporting Goods and buy some of the same balls just to make sure they perform the same as the ones the company submitted for testing.

The painstaking attention to detail does not end with the testing. Every person who submits an item, including something like the obviously nonconforming three-headed putter, receives a meticulously written decision after a committee of four meets. The submission has a file, including all the correspondence involved should the person want to appeal the decision, which is allowed (the appeal goes to a different committee). All the paperwork is kept on file, as are all the submitted items. More than 27,000 files are stored at the test center and kept confidential. I asked for a peek at all of these odd items when I visited there a few years ago. They led me away as if I were insane. Everybody's crazy, or not so crazy, notion of how to improve golf is sacrosanct. The mad golf scientist/basement lab tinkering that went into the building of the three-headed putter is as secret as the formula for Coca-Cola.

Is all of this scrutiny worth it? Well, I don't know about you, but it makes me feel safer knowing there is some golf sheriff watching over the Wild West–like landscape of golf products — just as there are men and women meticulously standing guard over every tenet and every word of the game's time-honored bylaws. It makes me feel as though I'm part of a distinct society. You become a golfer and you get all these noble, orderly, and imperative principles by which to abide. And that is vitally important for a game played by people in ugly shoes holding crooked sticks manically chasing a little white ball across a seemingly endless field.

So, yes, we have to have rules, I mean Rules. Because maybe there is some righteousness to golf, after all. Maybe there is some basic, over-arching fairness and justice.

Oh, who am I kidding? It's golf.

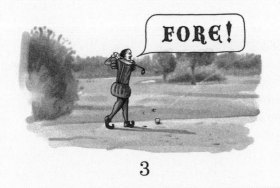

3

The Language of Golf

Golf is a game in which you yell fore,
shoot six, and write down five.

BROADCASTER PAUL HARVEY

DO YOU SPEAK golf?

Do you play for Barkies? Or Arnies? Do you avail yourself of the breakfast ball and love a good game of Bingo, Bango, Bongo?

Have you found yourself dormie, stymied, plugged, or in the cabbage?

Have you dubbed it, shrimped it, shanked it, dinked it, or duck-hooked it? And do you know the difference? Have you hit a scooter? How about one in the side door?

Are you a sandbagger? A pigeon? A player? A hooker?

Do you know who lovingly called his putter Billy Baroo?

In other words, are you conversant in the dialect of golf? Do you not only play golf but also revel in all of its idiosyncratic, peculiar lingo?

Indeed, it is the code of the tribe, sometimes the most convivial part of being in the weird golf fraternity. Nothing can assuage the misery of a poor shot like a good, self-deprecating idiom for your idiocy.

Golfers could say, "Oh, that's a bad shot." But why, when they can say they chunked it, skulled it, or smothered it?

And golf linguistics are not just for your bad shots. In fact, most of the terms deal with making fun of your partners' shots. Because theirs are never simply in trouble, in a pond, or out-of-bounds. They are in jail, rinsed, or Oscar Bravo.

This vernacular is centuries old, passed on and continually abridged and expanded. Some of it is amazingly relevant. There are sayings linked to Rush Limbaugh and Nancy Pelosi (think of shots going right or left), Osama bin Laden (think of all of the bunkers on a golf course), and Paris Hilton (think of anything). Some references are risqué or crude. There are a host of terms linked to dead people and a lot of sexual innuendo. You have to be careful what you say if playing with juniors or the easily offended. But it makes me feel good that golf — a so-called stodgy game invented five centuries ago — can stay current. We can use lingo that would be familiar to a golfer from 200 years ago. But we don't have to — golfers in the 1800s didn't have Viagra jokes.

It also proves to me something nongolfers often fail to grasp: Old-fashioned golf is at its heart an old-fashioned social exercise.

"Golf lingo developed because the golf course is a place where people get to know each other, and the game is so hard it especially leads to teasing, joking, and ragging on each other," said Randy Voorhees, the author of *The Little Book of Golf Slang*.

"The lingo has persisted because golf is a game you play for a lifetime," he said. "So parents pass the terms on to their children, or older players use this colorful vernacular around younger players, and it becomes a natural way of speaking on the golf course."

The first time you hit a ball on the green and someone calls for it to "sit," does that not perfectly describe what you want the ball to do? If you hit a ball into the water and someone says it is "wet," does that not forevermore seem like the best portrayal of its position and your disposition?

"A lot of golf terms actually evoke an image of what is happening out there," Voorhees said. "You can carve, feather, or gouge a shot, and once you learn to perform those shots, they are words that exactly describe what you're trying to do."

The golf lexicon has not developed by accident. David Normoyle, the assistant director of the United States Golf Association Museum, cited three primary reasons.

"One, golf is played over such a vast, irregular surface, we need a myriad of descriptions for play on a golf course," he said. "Two, golf is truly a global game and has many local variations and flavors. Last, and perhaps more than anything else, golf has had great poets, and they have tried to capture the essence of the game."

Who knew that having "the shanks" was meant to be literature?

The roots of our golf language are deep, and the words mark the passage of golf from fifteenth-century Scotland to England to France, back to Scotland and on to North America. And then back again. Like any dialect, some of it is provincial and some of it is understood only if you have an ear for the local accent or native tongue. Play with a Scottish caddie sometime, and on the first tee he might seem to be asking if you play "compost golf."

Now, that may not sound like a very neighborly question. Compost golf? As in dung? Manure golf? What are you saying?

It's not quite as bad as it sounds. He is asking if you play "compass golf." In other words, if he is going to accompany you for the day, will he need his compass to find his way back to the fairway or golf course?

That's actually pretty funny. Unless you really do have a compass in your bag.

Most golf terms are simpler, and we actually know quite a bit about them. Since being a golf historian combines two of humankind's most basic instincts — obsessing over something trivial (golf) and wasting time (researching trivia) — we know a lot about how most prominent golf terms came to be. Take, for example, the origin of the word *caddie*. Most golf historians, who when they aren't busy taking naps between the book stacks at ancient European libraries write long treatises on golf language, believe *caddie* derives from the French *le cadet*, meaning "the boy" or someone young. The word *cadet* began appearing in English writings around 1610. About twenty years later, *caddie* or *cadie* appeared in print to describe someone who carries the clubs for another golfer, usually one of greater social standing.

Some have surmised that military cadets started doing this for royalty or high-ranking officers. This might account for all the obsequious toadying some people have come to expect from their caddie. And that certainly was the image — and the practice — two generations ago.

The historical data on some of the most common golf jargon proves how quickly golf entwined itself in common culture, even 200 years ago. A *bogey* refers to the bogeyman, used in a popular British song. The bogeyman was more like a goblin or devil, but the idea was to catch him (if you can). And somehow chasing the perfect score in golf became chasing "bogey." That's right, a bogey score was good. Near the end of the 1800s, as "modern" materials and club making improved, golfers were getting better and shooting lower golf scores. A bogey round was no longer thought of as good enough.

The term *par,* which had been around for many years and meant "average" or "usual," came to connote the expected score for an expert golfer, while *bogey* became the expected score for a decent recreational golfer.

The use of *par* spread with golf's help. Stocks were soon rated as "on par" — where have I heard that term before? — or subpar. Other things were "par for the course."

Some terms seem silly now but made perfect sense at the time. Near the end of the nineteenth century, something described as "a bird" was something good or favorable. So people referred to a shot close to the hole as "a bird of a shot." In time, that became a birdie.

The bird theme continued to eagle and albatross (3 under par), and for a while some people called a double bogey a "buzzard." Three consecutive birdies became a turkey. Thankfully, the radio was invented and I'm thinking people spent less time hunched in arboretums with binoculars so golf wrested its dictionary away from the ornithologists.

Soon, we developed more throaty, audacious-sounding slang. We golfers were hackers, duffers, and sandbaggers. Well-struck shots were nuked and poor ones were jacked. We hit punch shots with our mashie club and mastered the knock-down approach. The terminology grew infinitely more clever:

A putt that won't go in the hole is afraid of the dark.

A putt that encircles the hole before it falls in takes a victory lap.

A putt that is unreadable is a Salman Rushdie.

Now, if you're a beginner or a casual player, you may find golfspeak to be another intimidating barrier to feeling comfortable on the course —a verbal version of golf behavioral etiquette. But don't fret.

There are no secret passwords in the pro shop or trick questions posed on the first tee. People are engrossed in their own games. Don't play slowly or throw your clubs, and no one will care much about your golf vocabulary.

"Keep your ears open; you'll learn it all as you go," Voorhees said. "Soon it will flow out of your mouth naturally."

It is how golf lingo evolved and continues to evolve. Why needle your partner by saying, "Hey, you hit it in the sand," when you can instead ask, "Got your sunscreen for the beach?"

And the next time he hits it in a bunker, you say: "Got your SPF 50? Because you could be there for a while."

Of course, it's not just about teasing or jabbing those with you. Golf slang unquestionably exists to diffuse our embarrassment about golf's unending assortment of bad shots. When you barely hit a short, easy chip, sending it no more than a few feet forward, either you can say you mishit it, or you can exclaim that you "chili-dipped" it. Whatever that means.

Most people have no idea where that term came from, but all serious golfers know what you mean. You messed up something simple. We have been there.

Actually, in his large book *The Historical Dictionary of Golfing Terms: From 1500 to the Present,* author Peter Davies writes that the term may refer to a feeble attempt to make a scooping action, like someone trying to dig a chip into chili dip.

I'm not sure this makes sense, because I can't see my sand wedge blasting through the beans, tomatoes, and guacamole. But here's the good news: Whenever you use this term again, you will be thinking about food, about appetizers, and maybe a cool late afternoon on a terrace somewhere — and not about that ridiculously simple little chip you just flubbed.

Chili-dipped, indeed.

If you are new to golf, or just new to golf lingo, I do suggest that you make sure to visit the local municipal golf course. A lot about golf can be learned there in general, but without question, it is where you will hear the richest, sauciest golf phrases.

It's also a good place to try out your contributions. And that's really the point. Please, don't be a mute out there. I have a golf buddy named Kevin who likes to scream strange, unconnected names at his ball if he hits a poor shot. He'll yell, "Oh, what a Betty!" as a ball is heading for the water. Next time, it might be "Are you kidding me? Such a Horace." Or "Give me a break, Cesar."

I prefer this to the golfers who when they strike a bad shot scold themselves in the third person and always with their given name, as if they were their mother watching from the porch:

"Oh, Thomas."

"Oh, Robert."

"Oh, Margaret."

"Oh, Thaddeus."

OK, so I've never played with a Thaddeus, at least that I'm aware of. But I'm sure it's happened on a golf course somewhere. It just figures that golf would be the game that makes us feel like we're once again eight years old, standing in short pants and getting lectured for doing something wrong.

But you don't have to feel that way. Break out the golf jargon. Shout something silly — "Nice shot, Fenton!"

Hey, you might come up with a new term for our treasured golf glossary.

Speaking of which, here is a summary of some of my favorite, most expressive golf slang. I'm leaving out most obvious terms and going for the rich, evocative ones:

Acey Deucey: A group betting game in which the low scorer on each hole (ace) wins money from the other three players and the high scorer (deuce) loses money to the other three players. This is meant to balance things out, but that works only if you aren't a recurring dunce, I mean deuce.

Aircraft carrier: A long, flat, rectangular teeing ground, one that is usually elevated above the fairway and includes all the tees for that hole. If you think about it, this is one of many golf terms meant to describe our unease on the golf course. Teeing off an imaginary aircraft carrier is no way to play with confidence. Where, after all, would the ball go if you hit it off an aircraft carrier?

Air mail: When you badly overshoot your target, usually the green. The ball flies too far, which will lead someone to tell you, "Really airmailed that green." The rejoinder? "Thanks; let's hope it's still in this ZIP code."

Army golf: You hit it left, right, left, right. Sound off! One, two, three, four. The score is adding up.

Barkie: A bet won for making par after hitting a tree.

Billy Baroo: References to the movie *Caddyshack* are sacred in the golf cult. The great Ted Knight, playing the character Judge Smails, called his lucky putter Billy Baroo. Years later, that commendation held such merit that it became the name of a line of real putters. If you are new to golf, understanding the Smails character's role in the American game is pivotal. Watch the movie some Saturday night after a great, or horrible, round. You'll feel better — and understand the lingo a bit better.

It also may help to explain why you've seen someone stand on the first tee and pause to announce, "Gambling is illegal at Bushwood, sir, and I never slice." Next time, you'll be able to bet a hundred bucks they slice it into the woods.

Bingo, Bango, Bongo: A points game in which a point is awarded for being the first player on the green (Bingo), for being closest to the hole when everyone has reached the green (Bango), and for being the first in the hole (Bongo). You'll be surprised how fast this makes sense.

Bo Derek: A score of 10 on any hole. But somebody needs to update this reference. Bo's movie *10* came out in 1979. I used this term once recently on the golf course and one of my younger partners said to me, "Did you say Bo Jackson?"

And then an even younger partner said, "Who's Bo Jackson?"

Cabbage: Deep or thick rough, as in "Took me three to get out of the cabbage." I'm not sure cabbage would actually be that hard to get out of, but it sounds hard.

Cat box: A bunker. The sand is like kitty litter, get it? Another rough image meant to make us play worse. But nonetheless, people like saying, "I found the cat box."

Chicken stick: A play-it-safe club choice. Instead of hitting a driver off the tee to a tight fairway, a chicken stick might be a 5- or 7-wood. This term is not always used admiringly. Your partner: "You gutless worm, I knew you'd go with the chicken stick."

Dawn patrol: Golfers who like to be the first ones on the course in the morning. Also known as **dew sweepers**.

Dog track: A golf course in poor shape or without much character, charm, or challenge. Dogs and cats are apparently not much admired in golf.

Duck hook: A shot that veers severely to the left for a right-handed golfer, or to the right for a lefty. It's more than a hook because it dives, or ducks, to the left (or right) immediately off the club. It has nothing to do with hitting ducks with the shot, though I have seen that happen because golf architects like to put little ponds near tee boxes. Ducks, which apparently have little golf acumen, will stand there hopelessly in harm's way of the nasty hook for which they are named.

Foot wedge: When players kick a golf ball into a better position because it is behind a tree, in the rough, or on a bare spot. This is also known as cheating, but when announced with a mischievous smile, the foot wedge comes off as more harmless in a face-saving sort of way.

Frog hair: The fringe or apron surrounding a green. Frogs do not have hair, but the term *frog hair* is actually a centuries-old simile that refers to something delicate. Like that terrifying side-hill chip you're going to have from the frog hair.

Hermie: A great, cross-cultural golf and TV reference. A Hermie is a very large divot, a term coined in tribute to the 1960s television character Herman Munster, who in one episode of *The Munsters* played golf and took rug-size divots. There was a movie remake of *The Munsters* but no new golf terms emerged from it.

Hosel takeover: The not-so-rare golf play on words. Another term for a **shank**.

Joe Pesci: A clever way to define a "mean, tough 5-footer." As in a short yet breaking downhill putt that could run 20 feet past the hole if missed. Pesci, the diminutive actor, often plays mean, tough guys. He's a pretty good golfer, as it happens. He probably doesn't fear mean 5-footers.

Linda Ronstadt: When one golfer out-drives another, as in Ronstadt's hit song "Blue Bayou." Get it? Blew by you. Surprisingly, this one term, *Linda Ronstadt*, endures even though Ronstadt hasn't had a hit song in decades.

Looping: It's another word for caddying. Looping just sounds much cooler.

Otis: A player who is terrific at getting up and down from any location. The "up" part means getting it on the green in one stroke. The "down" part means getting it down into the hole in one stroke. Always up and down, like an Otis elevator.

Saddam Hussein: When someone hits from a fairway sand trap to a greenside sand trap, he or she is going from bunker to bunker. This was a little funnier before Hussein was executed.

Scottish mulligan: It's not a do-over after a poor tee shot. It means you're hitting three.

Shank: A mishit where the club's hosel strikes the ball.

Star Trek **golf:** Going where no man has gone before. (I have also heard Trekkies refer to a shot that strikes the cart path as having gone **Carpathian**.)

A *Star Wars* **reference:** Not to be outdone, a ball is **Obi Wan** when it is out-of-bounds.

USA: Spoken after a partner's shot, it is meant to indicate that the partner is still away, as in "You shoot again."

U-turn: When the ball circles the hole and comes back at you without falling in the hole. This outcome often brings about other familiar golf terms: **#!%&@#)!$#!**

Now, these terms only scratch the surface when it comes to the realm of possible words a golfer uses to describe the game of golf. Consider, as one straightforward example, all the things that golfers yell at a ball as it is in flight:

"Get down"
"Hook"

"Grow teeth"
"Get up"
"Fade"
"Be the right stick"
"Bounce"
"Settle"
"Kick right"
"Kick left"
"Hit something"
"Hit a house"
"Run"
"Hop"
"Stop"
"Bite"
"Land like a butterfly with sore feet"

Yes, land like a butterfly with sore feet. I bet in the history of mankind those seven words have never been spoken anywhere but on a golf course. Who knows who started that? Let's get the golf historians on that one. Somebody go wake them up between the upstairs book stacks.

While we are waiting for an answer, we will all continue to say it.

The funny thing about golf lingo is that you have to leave room in your vocabulary for various descriptions of shots. It's not enough to have one bit of slang for a shot. And as I mentioned before, poor shots get special attention. They are always stabbed, cut, pulled, yanked, heeled, sprayed, skied, smothered, and thinned. Not surprisingly, less time has been spent on verbally depicting good shots, but we have some good words for them. Good shots are usually pured, flushed, crushed, cranked, nailed, or hit on the screws, even though our woods no longer have screws on the clubface. (Old persimmon-headed drivers had a clubface insert held in place by screws.)

But the enchanting thing about golf talk is that it is so much more than one-word sayings.

People run around greens happily declaring, "Never up, never in." What does that mean? I have no idea. At face value, it means that a putt that never gets up to the hole will never go in the hole. Which is a "no kidding" moment, and it may not even be good advice. Putts recklessly or overaggressively slammed so that they skitter 12 feet past the hole never go in either — plus you have a good chance of three-putting.

Give me "Never quite up but close enough for a tap-in" most of the time instead of "Never up, never in."

Here's another golf phrase I don't understand: "Trees are 90 percent air."

Well, even if we agree on that — a dubious assumption — I would make the point that a chain-link fence is also 90 percent air. Try hitting your ball through one.

But there are other popular golf phrases that are visually precise portrayals. A golfer who is thin is a "walking 1-iron." Not often used in groups of men over forty-five.

Someone who is a short hitter "can't hit it out of his shadow." Been there. It even happens late in the day.

Someone hitting it left and right is "shoelacing the course." I could weave my way through a Payless shoe store.

Facing a long 50-foot putt over a few humps and dips, a caddie might say: "That's a long camel ride."

I have been told by friends who are chemists that they refer to a ball that has landed in a body of water as "aqueous."

Yet another friend introduced me to the useful golf abbreviation LOIBIP. It stands for "Loss of Interest, Ball in Pocket." That perfectly describes one's attitude when you've already taken seven or eight swipes at the ball and now need to pick up and regroup mentally.

Everybody knows that an 8 on a hole is a snowman, but did you know that consecutive 8s is "piano keys"? As in 88?

And years ago, watching the British Open on television, I loved it when a putt would seem to be slowly slipping past the hole, only to suddenly topple in from the side. And the legendary British announcer Henry Longhurst would say, "Safely in the tradesman's entrance."

Even the pros have their own slang just for their world. A particularly bad shot late in the second round of a pro tournament is a "trunk slammer." Why?

Because that's the shot that makes the pro miss the tournament cut and get sent home for the weekend. Soon, he will be in the parking lot placing his clubs in the trunk so he can slam it in disgust and drive on down the road.

Some golf terms are draped in myth. No one seems to know why the approach shot that comes to rest closest to the pin at an outing or a tournament — a common, side-bet competition on a par 3 — is referred to as "KP," but people say it anyway. "The winner of the KP today is . . ."

It makes no sense, and I've asked around. Nobody knows where it came from. We say it anyway.

Maybe it's better that we don't know. It makes it easier to forget it ever happened. Because someone once told me that any driver, putter, set of clubs, or golf vacation won in a closest-to-the-pin contest should be declared on your income taxes. Maybe KP stands for "Keep Pretending" (you found it).

Some other golf terms are bathed in history, such as the explanation for why golfers yell "Fore" when a wayward shot might strike another golfer.

There are many theories for the use of "Fore" but no sure answer, even though this is a part of golf etiquette dating to the eighteenth century. Some people believe it is some kind of shortened version of "forewarned." Others say it has to do with the fore and aft of a ship, with those in front needing the warning and hence, "fore."

But the most widely accepted explanation has its roots in the British military. The armies of the 1700s would form ranks with the infantry positioned in front of the artillery guns. It was customary, before the artillery began firing, to shout, "Beware before." That way, the infantry could lie down to avoid the cannonballs. As golf grew in popularity, it is believed that soldiers brought the term to the game as a way to warn other players of incoming golf shots. And the term was eventually shortened.

It's also a lot easier than yelling, "Watch out, here comes my Precept Laddie ball!"

Yelling "Fore" is the kind of time-honored yet mysterious thing real golfers do. Like excitedly yelling at a ball to "Get up" and then almost as quickly begging it to "Sit down." It's as if we could communicate for hours on the golf course using nothing but golf slang.

We would be referring to fried eggs, breakfast balls, chops, and chili dips and not even be talking about food. Somebody could be inside the leather, which sounds tortuous, even semi-illegal, but in fact, it would be the most calming condition of all because a golfer inside the leather is granted a gimme. And doesn't a gimme sound cozy and snug?

The language of golf is limitless and defining at the same time, like the game itself but unto itself. Only golf could find such rich and varied ways to depict our pleasure and our misery. It is the game with its own tongue. It is how we speak golf. Swing away and let the lingo flow.

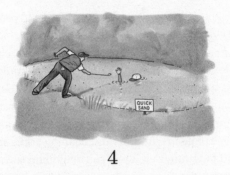

4

Being a Good Golf Partner
(and Surviving a Day with a Bad One)

Give me golf clubs, fresh air, and a beautiful partner,
and you can keep the clubs and the fresh air.

JACK BENNY

THERE WAS THE GUY who liked to make little clicking noises with his teeth as I was swinging. There was the guy who giggled when I missed a putt. There was the guy who removed his golf glove and then put it back on — twice — before and after every shot. Another guy wanted to bet on the outcome of every hole, and when that wasn't enough excitement, he started to propose bets on the outcome of each shot. There was the woman who drove her cart very fast, and frequently over my ball as it lay in the fairway. There was the guy who if he missed a putt — and he missed often — would remain on the green and try it again, not once, but three or four times. There was the guy who liked to give a long, detailed assessment of each of his shots just after he struck them:

"You know, I was trying to hit it left to right, but I caught it a little thin so it wouldn't fade. I've been working on firing my right side, but

I overrotated and my hands got behind me. Yeah, Tiger has the same problem I do. So that's why my ball bounced left and I'm in the short rough. I've got a new hybrid for those kinds of lies, though. Been practicing it with my backyard net. Do you have a backyard net? You gotta get a backyard net. My wife bought me one for Christmas. Well, not this Christmas, but two years ago on Christmas. We were in Bermuda. You ever been to Bermuda? No? You gotta play golf in Bermuda. The ocean air makes the ball fly farther. And you know, you could use the extra yardage. Yeah, I took a lesson there. That's where I learned to hit it left to right. But I caught it a little thin just now. Wouldn't fade. You know what I mean? You play a fade?"

One of the joys of playing golf is that you will meet a lot of different people. One of the inconveniences of playing golf is that you will meet a lot of *different* people.

A day on the golf course becomes memorable and cherished with the right partner. A day on the golf course becomes an interminable nightmare with the wrong one. I have had many more good golf partners than bad ones over the years. But the bad ones tend to stick with you longer, like a persistent grass stain you can't wash out of your khakis.

If you're going to play golf, a fundamental, central goal is to be a good partner to those around you. It is a responsibility you fulfill, and in return, it often becomes the reward you harvest. The great thing about golf is that it is usually a mix of individual pursuit and shared experience. You can play alone. You will eventually miss playing with others.

But golf changes in the company of others. Group golf is a game with a completely different rhythm and pace. It requires more sensibility, more awareness, and more consideration. It takes tact, empathy, and, especially, good humor. It is delicately, or robustly, social. It is amusing, unpredictable, and occasionally aggravating and embarrassing. But at its best, it can expand your commitment to and understanding of golf itself.

Group golf is like a two- or four-person raft trip down a choppy, rapid-filled river. The goal is for everyone to step from the raft unscathed and smiling at the end.

And then you go have a beer and pay off the bets.

But along the way, the people accompanying us on golf's ongoing journey, even if it is four random hours once and nevermore, become part of a golfer's continuous golf narrative. You may never see that golf partner again, but you will likely remember him or her for the place, for shots struck, or for odd or memorable things that happened. Occasionally, you will recall a partner for the wrong reasons, but there will also be memories of the most magnanimous gestures and graces.

Golf partners, including those we play with over and over, are fixtures in our personal golf stories, more lasting than a score registered or the discoveries of a new golf course played. It is not just the golf we played that day. It is the golf we shared that day.

This is true because golf, like other sports, was invented to be a game of more than one. The word *partner* appears on the first page of the Rules of Golf.

So the golf partner is a fundamental element of the game. We play with partners and we are all someone else's partner. On the face of it, being a good partner doesn't sound very complicated. All it takes is someone who generally gets along with others, right? This makes sense until you realize that golf can make people crazy.

There is another problem. Because golf is a web of passed-down protocols and etiquette going back centuries, with some habits developed in tense competition, it is easy for an otherwise well-intentioned golfer to unsuspectingly violate simple good golf manners. Next, there is the undeniable fact that keeping your equilibrium through four or five hours on the golf course is considerably harder than acting normal at a cocktail party or a wedding. Golf will put everyone toting a bag through a long series of pressure-filled tasks. On a golf course, even the dignified and studiously unruffled can be reduced to wild fits of club throwing. Finally, the world is not entirely filled with gracious and courteous people. And sometimes the situation itself, like when you are on vacation and playing as a single, can bring out an altogether new set of circumstances that require diplomacy and patience.

Being a good partner also touches on two incandescently contentious golf issues: slow play and playing from the appropriate tees. Each will be mentioned early in this chapter and explored in full later. But first, let's emphasize what everyone can do to make the day more pleasant — for you and your partners. There are common mistakes and misbehaviors, and I have been guilty of all of them at one time or another in my golf life. So to get everyone teed off on the subject — get it? — here are the ten most annoying things people do on the golf course:

10. They stand in another player's line of sight.

It's pretty simple: Stand where you can see either the chest or the backbone of the person hitting, preferably the backbone if on the tee. Anywhere else can be a distraction. That especially includes the putting green. For example, don't stand behind the hole as someone putts. As we putt and stare at the hole in preparation, we don't want our attention diverted to the fact that you have mismatched socks or an unzipped fly.

9. When they shank a shot, they immediately pull another ball from their pocket and hit a do-over.

This often happens several times a round, holding everyone else up. Worse, they usually shank the second shot as well.

8. They play from the wrong tees, usually the back or championship tees.

New equipment technology has casual players thinking they can drive the ball 275 yards just because it happened once — on the range. Statistics show that the average golfer usually hits a driver less than 210 yards. Problem is, the vast majority of people never think of themselves as average. So the tees that are farthest away, once actually reserved for championships, are jammed full of players insisting on "seeing the whole course."

More on this counterproductive and increasingly routine custom later. For now, it's important to realize that golf is not a pie-eating contest. More is not better; it just makes you and everyone else take longer to play a round.

7. They act as if they were Rules mavens.

We've established the necessity of the Rules, but we don't need anyone loudly and officiously castigating some novice player for innocently breaking Rule 18-2, because the player's ball moved slightly after a practice swing. Some people are just learning or simply out to play a friendly round. A quiet conversation later about some Rules would suffice.

6. They make excuses after bad shots.

Golf is a fickle game. Unfair things happen out there. But it is better to take it in silence. I have done the opposite, and I swear that if you whine, the golf gods will make it worse. Picture two clubs in a tree.

It is tempting to point out the unjust, incomprehensible things that can happen. How do you explain a shot that skirts all the big, imposing trees in your line but then deflects off a tiny branch and drops down onto a cart path that then ricochets your ball into a pond? You'll want to screech and howl, especially since it always seems to happen right after your partner's ball skips three times across the same pond and rolls safely onto the green. But just as you must bite your tongue when your boss says something exceptionally stupid, and just as you don't take sides when two of your crazed in-laws get into an argument, remaining mum is the best choice of inaction.

Everyone else will see that an unlucky, or just plain bad, shot happened. Take that misfortune with grace and one of the truly rare things in golf might happen: Someone will feel sorry for you.

5. They are oblivious to other golfers, walking through the rough yelling, "Hey, did you see my ball?" just as someone else in the foursome is preparing to hit.

It is better to know what is going on around you and respect your surroundings. Don't just pull the cigar out of your mouth and scream, "Found it!" Even if your foursome isn't bothered, someone on an adjacent tee might be. It's all right to be loud sometimes, such as when a 50-foot birdie putt rolls over hill and dale and falls in the hole. But boisterously tramping around from hole to hole shouting out instructions or drink orders ruins the atmosphere all around you.

I understand, we're out there to have fun. True, a golf round isn't a prayer service — even with all the praying going on — but it's not a rodeo either. Although I admit that the occasional clown in a barrel might loosen things up after a tough par 5.

4. They cheat.

We've covered much of this territory before. But when it comes to being a good golf partner, it's important to act like you respect the game. Don't roll your ball over to a better lie in the fairway unless you know the course is playing winter rules or someone else in the group has declared that kind of thing acceptable. Don't rake away every 3-foot putt as if it's a gimme unless your partner gives you the putt. You don't have to be a stickler for the Rules; just don't take advantage of them. Why does this matter? Because your partners will notice and probably talk about you later. It's not worth it. Golf gossip is worse than middle-school gossip, and it definitely sticks to you longer.

3. They take too many practice swings.

I know you've seen Phil Mickelson take four or five practice swings on the eighteenth tee of a big tournament. Or maybe you just took a lesson, and you're working on something. But the rest of us had hopes of getting to our cars before David Letterman starts his monologue. Take one practice swing, at most. Chances are, you will play better. This is also part of the slow play problem, so more on that later.

2. They brag about their equipment.

If you are an 18 handicap but you genuinely feel you must play with blade irons or you swing too hard to use those "too-soft" graphite shafts, there's no rule against such illusions. But the rest of us don't have to be introduced to your dream world.

This also goes for explanations about why you play the Pro V1x ball instead of the Pro V1. No one wants to hear about the spin rates you say you impart with your short irons. We have noticed that your Pro V1x sinks in most ponds at roughly the same rate as the standard Pro V1 you used to play.

1. They use their cell phones.

This is, without question, the most annoying, irritating thing of all and the unquestioned bane of the golf course. Cell phones should be turned off, and if you must check into the digital world, be discreet and tactful. Turning your back to the green as you talk on the phone doesn't qualify. It just makes your partners make faces behind your back. Don't we go to the golf course to enjoy the outdoors and be away from the office? So why do so many people spend sixteen of eighteen holes immersed in their smartphone as they ignore the outdoors and the pleasures of golf?

So those are the things that annoy. What are the things that separate a good partner from a bad one? Here are ten tips for being the golf partner others remember for all the right reasons:

1. Be on time.

We're all busy and it's easy to be a little tardy, but don't add to the apprehension that plagues every first tee by making your partners wonder if you're going to be there on time. First impressions matter in golf as much as elsewhere in life, so be the considerate one who is ready to go. It's a small thing that goes a long way to getting everyone off on the right foot.

2. Be quiet.

When someone else is standing over the ball preparing to hit, that's not the time to suddenly check your pockets for your car keys. Don't adjust the Velcro on your golf glove or scrape dirt off your sand wedge with your putter. Stand still, and unless a blimp is about to crash on the course, don't move. And please, don't whisper to the person next to you, because you are heard.

3. Know when to speak up and what to say.

This is a little trickier.

"The emotions of every golf outing ebb and flow throughout the day," Laird Small, the director of instruction at the Pebble Beach Golf Academy, told me years ago. "I tell my students that it's in their best interests to keep their partners in a positive frame of mind. So be optimistic. When somebody hits something a little crooked, say something nice like 'You really struck that well — just missed it a little.'

"Or say, 'You can get up and down from there.' Try to get them thinking about the next shot."

The point is to put yourself in the other golfer's shoes. And try to keep things light.

I was once playing a short par 3 over water with Lee Trevino at a charity outing and proceeded to hit a screaming line drive that never got more than 2 feet off the ground — until it disappeared in the very front of the pond.

Trevino said, "Wow, Bill, that's the straightest shot you've hit all day." I was still embarrassed but I was laughing.

4. Mind the flagstick.

This is not a little thing, though it may seem so. If your ball is the closest to the hole when you reach the green, pull the flag for the group because you are going to be the last to putt anyway. Or if you get to the green first, grab the flag.

You have the same responsibility if you have putted out; look for the flag so others don't have to. It gets on people's nerves if you treat the flag as always somebody else's problem. And be careful where you put the flagstick after you've taken it from the hole. Assess each person's possible putting line, including the likelihood that some putts will be poorly struck — hey, I've seen your foursome. So don't put the flag somewhere that might interfere with a wayward putt. No one will think that's funny. Put the flag where it cannot be in play.

If you are the one putting the flagstick back in the hole, also be careful. It's very easy to miss the center of the hole and damage the grass on the edges. This can lead to lipped-out putts for golfers playing after you. So as a courtesy, keep the hole in perfect shape. Besides, you don't want to be the cause of that kind of bad karma. It will come back to haunt you.

5. Watch the flight of everyone's shots.

Your job on the golf course is not to simply focus on your own game. Keep your head up and keep an eye on what your partners are doing. Everyone needs the help because we all hit wayward shots. There is also some safety involved — your own safety. I have seen people hit by golf balls on the golf course and it sometimes isn't pretty. Often, the person who gets hit has not been paying attention to what a playing partner is doing and wanders into harm's way. Keeping up with everyone's game keeps you out of the line of fire.

6. Help others look for lost balls.

The golf tribe is not exactly a collection of Lewis and Clarks. We get lost all the time. A good partner gets out of the cart and tromps around looking for that hard-to-find little orb. A major tip for this exercise: Almost all golfers think their shots travel farther than they really do. So while your partner might be looking in the rough 200 yards down the fairway, you should turn back and start checking at the 170-yard mark. Then walk forward. Walking is the best way to look, by the way. Some things can be done from the cart, but if you keep circling in the vehicle, you're probably going to run over the ball. That will really make your partner happy.

So get out and lend a fellow duffer a hand. On the other hand:

7. Don't make everyone look for your ball for ten minutes.

According to the Rules, you have five minutes to find a lost ball. But if you hit your ball so far into the woods that you would need a miner's cap to find it, don't waste everybody's time. And remember, hit a provisional ball before you go to look. That way, no one waits as you go back to the tee to reload.

8. Maintain a good attitude regardless of how you're playing.

If things are going badly, there's no sense spreading the tension of your lousy round throughout the group. This, of course, applies to throwing clubs or overdoing the obscenities, but silent protests can cast a pall, too. If you go mute or start stamping around because you just triple-bogeyed two consecutive holes, you will put everyone on edge. So yes, you're upset; the best thing to do is change the subject.

Ask your partners about their jobs or their families. Ask why they play that particular brand of ball. Think of something, anything — How 'bout them Cowboys? Why does the American League use the designated hitter? Why is there Braille on the buttons for drive-through ATMs?

Anyone can be chatty and comfortable when things are going well. If you become a different person when things are going poorly, not only will it be more difficult to find your way back to the chatty and comfortable guy, but when you do start playing well and try to reconnect with your partners, they'll give you a look that says, "Oh, sure, now you want to talk."

It's not worth it. Everyone goes through bad stretches. Try to ride it out with good humor.

9. Avoid giving unsolicited advice.

Nobody likes a know-it-all. Even if you've got a good tip to share, your partner is going to be really steamed at you if it doesn't work out.

"The golf course in the middle of a round is no place to start working on a new swing," Butch Harmon, a coach to many of the best players in the last twenty-five years, once told me. "Play with what you got that day. Seek help later."

And if you still can't resist giving advice, remember this: It's also against the Rules.

10. Be generous, be honest, be nice.

Be generous with praise, because it's a hard game and we all need a boost. Be generous at the beverage cart — don't buy drinks and snacks just for yourself. Be honest about your score. Swallow hard and admit you made a 9. Be honest about your handicap. Don't say, "I'm about a 16." Give an accurate number. Be nice; compliment people on their wardrobe or their golf bag. Smile a lot, as if you are enjoying yourself. It will be infectious.

These are not the only things that good partners do. Good golf partners also do little chores for the people they play with, such as examining each green as they leave it to make sure no one has left a wedge on the apron. That happens a lot. You will save your playing partners at least one club per eighteen holes and they will thank you for it. A good partner also has an extra tee in his or her pocket, if not an extra ball. It comes in handy. And a good partner might rake the sand for you if it helps to speed play.

Because we all hate slow play.

Slow Play, the Scourge of Modern American Golf

Now we're really getting to the crux of being a good partner. Slow play is killing golf, and being the slowest in your group is the surest way not to be invited back for another round. Even if you follow all of the aforementioned courtesies, if you are interminably slow, there are not many golfers out there who will put up with you.

How has American golf gotten so slow? It's fair to start with the golf we watch on television. Pro golfers take way too long to hit every shot and have elaborate pre-shot routines that, unfortunately, I fear average golfers emulate. This has led to almost everyone taking one or two or three too many practice swings before every shot. I don't know how this has become so commonplace. Twenty-five years ago, when a four-hour round was considered somewhat long, not many people took any practice swings except before putts, and even that wasn't universal. Or there might be one practice swing per hole per player. Nowadays, it's not unusual for the average foursome to collectively take twenty practice swings per hole, including mindless swipes on the putting surface. You don't believe me? Try counting the warm-up swings on a hole sometime. It's astounding. And it helps to explain why the average recreational golf round now takes five hours or more to complete.

Slow play is more than too many practice swings. The causes are assorted. People fixate on getting the correct yardage, another thing we may have learned from watching the pros. Pre-shot routines include more than practice swings; sometimes there are various waggles, restless foot positioning, and breathing exercises that resemble a Lamaze class. This process keeps getting longer even though almost everyone agrees that average golfers would all play better if they played faster. But most of us can't seem to pick up the pace.

In fact, a surprising amount of research has been conducted in an effort to understand the epidemic of slow play, and there are now numerous theories about how to cure it. The easiest thing to do is watch faster players, like our recreational brethren in the United Kingdom, and see what they do differently. For example:

- They assess their upcoming shot as others in the group are assessing theirs. So they have calculated the distance, picked a club, and are ready to go within fifteen seconds of the last shot struck.
- They leave their cell phones in the car. The anti-phone diatribe bears repeating.
- They start reading a putt as soon as they reach the green. Too many slow players don't even look at their putt until it is their turn. Unless you're putting first, there's ample time to see your putt's line as others are putting. Then, when it's your turn, you're almost ready to go.
- They don't mark lagged putts. Especially if it is relatively short, you should just go ahead and putt out.
- They walk, which, contrary to the general wisdom, is usually faster. But if they do take a cart, they aren't afraid to hustle to where a partner has driven the cart. Driving the cart back and forth to pick up players adds time to a round.

Now, it's also true that slow play is not entirely the fault of the player. "Slow golfers are only half the equation when it comes to slow play," Bill Yates, the founder of Pace Manager Systems, a California company that consults with hundreds of golf courses about speeding play, says.

"The other half is the management of the golf course." The number one thing those running golf courses can do, Yates said, is space out tee times so the course won't be overcrowded. People often end up waiting not because golfers are playing slowly, but for the same reason traffic bogs down at rush hour. The golf courses can't handle the increased flow. Golf course owners may say that they make more money by having more golfers tee off more often, but Yates countered that an overburdened course keeps players waiting — and leaving unhappy, perhaps not to return to that course again.

"It's better business to provide a smooth experience around the golf course," Yates says. His advice, however, can become more complicated. For example, he says that blind landing areas and high rough on the inside of a dogleg are documented pace-of-play killers because they lead to waves of golfers looking for errant shots. Also, modern ball and club technology has led to longer golf courses, and longer holes take longer to play. Many resorts and high-priced private clubs have also added prodigious length to their designs. It's become a yardage arms race: The once-rare 7,000-yard course is now 7,500 yards, and 8,000 yards is coming to a resort near you. Magazines that rate golf courses fuel the madness by recognizing the behemoths as something special. And here's the worst part. You know what happens when you add tee boxes that stretch the holes to outrageous distances?

Scores of people want to play from them. They are supposed to be championship tees for elite players, but average and below-average golfers flock to them in some kind of rite of passage. And that slows play more than any other thing recreational golfers do.

Several years ago, Pete Dye, the mad scientist of golf architecture, was showing me around one of his new layouts. When I noticed that the most challenging tees, the ones farthest from the holes, were often obscured by landscaping, trees, or other natural terrain elements, Dye smiled mischievously and said, "That's to hide them from the ding-a-lings who don't belong there."

"We love our pro tees," Dye said, "but too many non-pros march back there. Then they wonder why they're not having fun."

If you play golf just about anywhere in the United States, you know the blight of the game is the groups of men — and it is almost universally men — playing from back tees that are way beyond their skill level. They're called the tournament tees. Employees at golf courses call them the testosterone tees.

People who insist on playing the most challenging tees always have a reason:

"I want to see the whole course."

"I want my money's worth."

"Playing from the back is the only way to compare myself to pro golfers."

"It's the only way to get better."

These are well-intentioned excuses or selfish ones. The real reason people keep playing from the wrong tees is that charming little golf defense mechanism I mentioned earlier, the one that keeps us playing at all. We as golfers think we are far better than we actually are. It's the only way to survive the truth of this merciless game. So we may acknowledge that studies have shown that the average male golfer hits his drive less than 210 yards, but thank goodness most of us aren't that average. A typical drive by a woman measures in the 125- to 140-yard range. Women, the same studies confirm, are less likely to overestimate that distance when asked.

So it is some combination of ego, peer pressure, and self-deluding miscalculation that keeps people marching farther and farther away to start each hole. And again, listing a gaudy set of tees on the scorecard that measure to 7,700 yards is like wheeling the dessert tray past a table of twelve-year-olds.

"There's another factor," said Joe Hallett, the former director of the PGA Center for Golf Learning and Performance in Port St. Lucie, Florida. "New technology does make the ball go farther, and that gets in people's heads. But if you go to the back tees hole after hole, you have to try to hit a home run every time up. And with that mindset you're going to hit some foul balls.

"Even when you do hit it straight, you'll probably have a hybrid in your hand every hole. What fun is that?"

And if you don't hit it straight and long, you'll be chipping out of the rough fronting the fairway or from the woods on the left or right, and then you'll still have a hybrid or a long iron to the green. Obviously, it's also simple logic that scores rise as holes lengthen. More strokes means more time on each hole, backing up the entire course.

Golf course designers have confronted this predicament by installing five or six sets of tees, with lengths beginning at 3,500 yards. Often, they have cleverly eliminated the traditional blue-white-red/back-center-front tee designations and substituted colors and shades that are not easily identified — or stigmatized. If the tees are black, oak, granite, orange, and green, the only reasonable way to choose what tees to play is to ask for help in the pro shop, or from the starter. Women aren't automatically sent to the red "ladies" tees; men might be persuaded to move forward a bit.

When Denny Perry was building the Harbor Rocks Golf Club in the lush hills of Virginia's Shenandoah Valley in 2002, he installed huge tee boxes for six sets of tees that play from 3,800 to 7,200 yards. The Harbor Rocks pro shop devised a chart to guide people: If you're a 26 to 30 handicap, head to the yellow tees, which play about 4,770 yards. If you're a 19 to 25, head to the orange (5,400 yards), and so on. You need permission from the pro shop to play the back tees (7,151 yards). I've played Harbor Rocks, and there are many forced carries and water hazards off the tee. Their advice was a godsend.

"Sometimes, we'll have a group struggling and playing slow and we'll suggest they move up a set of tees," Perry said. "A lot of them will come into the pro shop afterward to thank us. One guy said: 'I was ready to give up golf. Then I started having fun.'"

One problem with using handicaps to choose the appropriate tee is that fewer than a quarter of all golfers have one. So golf course architects, teaching pros, and recently the USGA and the PGA of America have proposed formulas instead. They work. But will golfers accept the number they are assigned?

One formula has a golfer estimate the average distance that his or her 5-iron shot will travel — an honest average, not the ultimate 5-iron — and then multiply that number by 36. If golfers were realistic, that would put most in the 5,300- to 6,300-yard range. Beginners, younger players, some seniors, and some women would play from tees more forward and be challenged. And the rare golfer, usually with a handicap in the low single digits, would be venturing back.

Another way to look at it: Assess the course's scorecard beforehand and find what looks like a typical par 4 — not the longest and not the shortest. From what tee will you be left with no more than a 7-iron to the green if you hit your driver its *average* distance? And if you seem to fall between two sets of tees and can't decide — since many golf courses don't do a good enough job advising people on this choice — you should play the shorter of the two tee offerings.

The USGA and PGA of America's "Tee It Forward" initiative includes a chart for picking the right tees. It is based on how far you hit your driver on average (again, honesty and modesty are key):

> Drive of 275 yards, play from tees measuring 6,700 to 6,900 yards
> Drive of 250 yards, play from 6,200 to 6,400 yards
> Drive of 225 yards, play from 5,800 to 6,000 yards
> Drive of 200 yards, play from 5,200 to 5,400 yards
> Drive of 175 yards, play from 4,400 to 4,600 yards
> Drive of 150 yards, play from 3,500 to 3,700 yards
> Drive of 125 yards, play from 2,800 to 3,000 yards

If this chart were used properly, most male golfers would be playing from tees that measure about 5,600 yards. Most women would be playing from tees that measure less than 3,700 yards.

There is one last rule of thumb that applies well to this situation, and it is elementary and easy to remember, too. If you aren't consistently breaking 90, move up one tee box until you are.

When I played golf with Dye in 2008, he didn't ask which tees I wanted to play but immediately walked to a set that would play about 6,000 yards. Truthfully, I promise, that's a little short for me using most measures. Dye occasionally took me back to the tournament tees for a gander. They were fearsome. Dye, eighty-two years old at the time, shot an 81; I was a few strokes back. It was a tough, tricky course that did not need length to give me fits. Walking off that eighteenth green, he still had that mischievous grin.

Playing from the wrong tees, and the slow play it can cause, is also a culprit of a little-discussed dark side issue for golf. I've taken to calling it golf rage. I have a Google alert set for the word *golf,* and it informs me about all kinds of things. But nothing in my golf Google alerts has shocked me like the stories of fisticuffs, shoving matches, assaults, and gunplay on the golf course — incidents often brought on by slow play.

Here's a small cross section of true-life situations:

In 2010, a thirty-three-year-old Seattle-area golfer was convicted of assault for hitting another golfer in the head with a 6-iron. The victim had been complaining about slow play on the golf course. The man wielding the 6-iron had been playing ahead of him.

Near Dallas the same year, a golfer was arrested on charges that he chased and punched a golfer playing behind him because the player hit a shot that ricocheted off his golf cart.

In England, also in 2010, a golfer was convicted of striking another golfer with an 8-iron because he thought the victim had hit his ball.

In Connecticut, a woman playing with her husband sustained permanent damage to her right eye when she was struck with a golf ball thrown by a man playing behind her. The man had been complaining about the pace of play, and on the eighteenth hole he walked forward and flung his golf ball at the woman. The man's playing partner approached the woman's husband and, after a brief argument, punched the husband in the head.

Admittedly, these are extreme cases, but they are not isolated events. Not only that, these are only the incidents that led to an arrest and made local news. Think of all the arguments, confrontations, and ugly moments that don't escalate and thus go unreported.

Talk to the staff at any pro shop, particularly at public courses, where the vast majority of American golf is played, and they will tell you it's common on busy weekends for someone to have to ride out to a distant hole to quell a budding disturbance. It's usually smoothed over, but the point is that people are getting a little riled up. And it is not always about slow play. Any number of things set people off. The stories are not much different from the ones you read about road rage. Except that it is different. This is golf. It's a game.

You stick a tee in the ground and an MMA bout breaks out? Isn't it hard enough to hit the ball?

I suppose it's no laughing matter, but a little recognition of the absurdity of it all may be helpful. As golfers, we are often wearing ridiculously bright-colored shirts. On our feet are some of the goofiest-looking shoes this side of the circus. We're hitting a tiny ball with insanely crooked sticks. And this is the moment we choose to defend our manhood?

How can this setting ever lead to blows? It seems more ripe for a barbecue. The only way golf course confrontations would make sense is if there were grandstands by the holes and nongolfers regularly came by to heckle us for being dumb enough to play this game.

OK, I won't joke anymore. This is a real, and growing, problem. When my file on these confrontations became an inch thick, I called around and talked to some experts, who offered explanations of the psychological and sociological origins of the rage. They also offered advice on how to prevent an incident, which might be beneficial someday.

Here is a summary of golf rage observations, even if some are obvious:

- Golf is frustrating, making people a little touchy.
- Many municipal golf courses are overcrowded, which makes it easier to accidentally interfere with someone else.
- Many new golfers have not been schooled in golf etiquette and do not realize that the behavior codes were developed to avoid confrontations and accord respect to everyone on the course. (They haven't read this book.)
- Alcohol plays a role in many of the most violent golf rage incidents.
- While there is a lot of slow play, people often erroneously blame the group directly in front of them when the problem is frequently a group three holes ahead. The slow play, in fact, could be coming from anywhere.
- But the most commonly cited cause of golf course altercations is primal. It comes down to territory and ego.

Joe Parent, the author of *Zen Golf* and *Golf: The Art of the Mental Game,* had this reaction:

"If someone hits into you while you're standing in the middle of the fairway, it's taken as a personal affront, since you were minding your own business. So you might say to yourself, 'I'm not backing down.' And you yell something. The guy behind you is thinking, 'Who's this guy? I'm not backing down, either.' Now it's a macho thing. It can escalate pretty quickly.

"People also look for scapegoats for their failures, and there are a lot of things that can go wrong on the course. So if someone on the adjacent hole yells during your backswing, you see him as the cause of your bad shot and you take that personally. You may feel compelled to tell him that he ruined your shot. In fact, you shouldn't take it so personally. It wasn't about you at all. That guy just likes to yell, and you got in the way."

Gregg Steinberg, who wrote *Mental Rules for Golf,* said that average golfers lack the emotional control of top players. This leads to outbursts.

"Everyone sees Tiger Woods or some other pro get mad on the golf course, but do they notice how quickly Tiger or the other player comes back to a calmness that allows him to concentrate on the next shot?" Steinberg said. "Most golfers have a pre-shot routine but need a post-shot routine, too. If you hit a bad shot, give yourself a few seconds to figure out what happened. You need that release. But don't overanalyze it. Say to yourself, 'Next shot,' and move on with a clear mind."

Parent, who is an instructor to many PGA Tour and LPGA Tour players, noted that in some European countries, golfers are required to get a golf license before they can play. He was not advocating such a policy, but licensing programs do ensure that new players know the basic good-conduct rules before they play. Junior golf programs in the United States, like the First Tee, do the same. Knowing the protocols outlined in this chapter will help you avoid unintended miscues and help you act like an experienced golfer who respects the movements of others on the golf course. As I've shown, it's not a lot of pomp and circumstance. It helps us all get around the golf course without annoying one another — too much.

A less noticed sidelight to the golf rage topic is damage to the golf course that overly angry golfers cause. We've all seen them, guys who bury a 5-iron in the tee box grass after a dribbled shot or deface the green after a poor putt.

"I tell people to be a little more accepting of the vagaries of golf and look at the big picture," Parent said. "What did you come out to the golf course for? To relax and have fun? Or to throw clubs? They want to play well, but they're missing the point.

"People think if they play better, they will enjoy it more. In reality, if they enjoy it more, they will play better."

Now, that's well said.

Vacation Golf

OK, so you've studied hard to become a good golf partner. You understand why it is so important. You'll never jiggle coins in your pocket on the teeing ground, you don't make excuses or talk on your cell phone, and you've learned to play fast. You're a skilled connoisseur of the recreational golf experience, learning as you go. You've been a good student. Are you ready for the final exam?

Because nothing will test you like a round of vacation golf. I'm not talking about buddy golf trips or beautiful sojourns to Ireland. I'm talking about slipping away by yourself for a round while at the beach, at the lake, or while visiting the in-laws. I'm talking about how once a year you pull up to a course you have never seen, play with people you have never met, pay a lot of money to do it, and then find yourself 11 over par after three holes.

Try making something fun out of that day, especially with a 9:00 a.m. tee time so that it's too early to start drinking.

It can be done. As a longtime sportswriter, I have played a lot of this vacation golf — OK, I was out of town working, but most games are at night so what else was I going to do during the day? Let me lead you on a typical day of vacation golf. You'll see the path and the lessons gained. In some ways, it's learning to be the ultimate golf partner.

Let's start in the pro shop, where you arrive after fifteen harried minutes spent looking for the tiny sign directing you to Creek Palms

Desert Island Dunes Ranch Spa, Resort, and Golf Club. The woman behind the desk points through the window to the range and says, "You're playing with those two gentlemen."

You look down and see two guys working on some kind of swing tip that involves one of them being on his back so he can tee the ball in his mouth. As you watch for another minute, you notice that they haven't paid for range balls. Instead, they're walking 30 yards into the range, ducking shots as they go, to gather topped balls so they can bring them back to the practice tee.

You decide to warm up on the putting green, which turns out to be the slowest surface you have ever stepped foot on. It feels as if you're putting through a bowl of soup. On the first tee, you meet your playing partners, Andy and Bob. You propose a friendly little betting game.

"What's your handicap?" you ask.

Andy pauses — always a bad sign — then mumbles, "Ah, maybe about . . . I don't know, 18 or 19?"

Bob turns to Andy and says: "What do you think I am? A 25?"

After you state your handicap, both of theirs go up two more strokes.

You survive the first-tee jitters, and the fact that Bob almost hit you with his tee shot even though you were standing even with the ball and to his right, and you end up with a par putt on the first green. Mindful of the practice surface, you give the ball a solid smack, and it rockets across the fastest green you've ever seen, rolling 30 yards back into the fairway.

"Geez, why'd you do that?" Andy says. "Everybody knows Creek Palms Desert Island Dunes Ranch has the fastest greens in the state."

You settle down for a handful of holes, making a few pars. Andy and Bob are busy giving each other advice and uttering inane golf sayings like "Trees are 90 percent air" as their shots ricochet through the woods. But at least they are playing quickly, and you've been pushing the group in front of you all day. Then, as you wait on the tee of a par 3, the group in front turns and waves for you to hit to the green.

Alas, it's one of the most feared and difficult shots in golf: Hit into the group you've been bugging and do it on a tricky par 3 as everyone watches and waits in judgment. Neither Andy nor Bob can get his ball airborne, and you skull a line-drive missile that nearly decapitates a woman in the foursome ahead of you even though she is standing 20 yards from the green. Your shot crashes into her cart, bounces around for a while, and comes to rest spinning inside one of their drinks in a cup holder.

"Look, a hole in one," you say with a forced smile when you reach their cart thirty seconds later. But no one is laughing. So what's the protocol? Do you pluck the ball out of the mint julep?

You drop another ball, play out as fast as you can, and scamper in shame to the next tee.

"Boy, I can't believe you almost killed the mayor's wife," Andy says.

"Yeah," Bob adds, "and the police chief and his wife didn't look too happy either."

But you have reached the halfway house after nine holes, and the food offerings are not the usual hot dogs or plastic-wrapped turkey sandwiches. They have barbecue sandwiches and an interesting-looking pickled something or other that spurs your adventurous side. Hey, it's vacation. And what do you know? It tastes good.

You tee off again, and your drives start to soar down the fairway, 10 or 15 yards farther than usual.

"That's the altitude," Andy says. "We're at 1,800 feet here, you know."

"No, it's the humidity," Bob counters. "Hydrogen-dominated water molecules replace nitrogen and oxygen in the air, making it lighter and therefore producing less friction, or drag, on a moving object, like a golf ball."

"It's the altitude, Bob. Lower atmospheric pressure at higher elevation. Everybody knows heavy, sticky air slows the ball down."

"It only feels heavy because the sweat evaporation cycle of the epidermis is slowed. The air is actually less dense."

You start to be intrigued by your new friends, especially since you keep winning holes as they keep stopping the cart person for refreshments. Andy and Bob are giving you tips about local, hidden-gem restaurants and telling charming, funny stories about the area. Or do they seem funny because you've stopped the beverage cart twice?

You're putting together some good shots now. You've even made two birdies. It's kind of fun playing with strangers instead of your usual partners, who know too well your weaknesses and golfing peccadilloes. When you hit into a particularly deep bunker on the sixteenth hole, no one cackles to remind you how poor a sand player you are. With a clear head and the belief that this out-of-town sand understands you better, you get up and down for par.

It's a beautiful day, the back nine is lush, and each sweeping view is new to your eye. There's wildlife by the ponds, not a cloud in the sky, and it's relaxing to saunter around, just waiting to see what's around the bend on each hole. You finish with the feeling that this was time well spent and exchange phone numbers with Andy and Bob.

OK, so you get lost leaving Creek Palms Desert Island Dunes Ranch, but that doesn't bother you. You'll find your way. Discovering and embracing the unknown seems to be part of the day's message. Although as you drive you are haunted by a question, like an eternal, unanswerable quandary: Altitude or humidity?

I told you every golf partner sticks with you somehow. It is part of the shared experience. Golf in tandem is a better game, and a good golf partner becomes as valued as a trusty, favorite club. We all strive to be that trusty partner. It is like striving to be a good friend. And if you believe as I do that there is something to be learned from every golf round, the lesson of good partnership is a lesson of selflessness.

It is an investment of self. Become a good partner and others will want to play with you again. There is an ultimate payout to that, besides invitations to play more often. You are creating good golf karma, and there is no doubt that good karma leads to good golf.

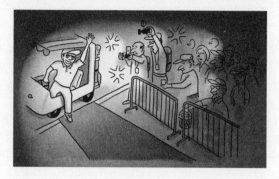

5

You're Not Alone Out There

*Golf can be humbling and will sometimes make you
feel pretty lonely out there; that's why they put
a big clubhouse behind the eighteenth hole.*

BYRON NELSON

ONE GUY SPLIT the seat of his pants on the first tee. Bill Hancock quietly mended the breach, and stifled the embarrassment, with the safety pins he always keeps handy.

Another guy, a newlywed, lost his wedding band somewhere before the first tee. Hancock found it on the practice range.

Two women pulled Hancock aside near the first tee and asked to be grouped with decent golfers who did not talk loudly. Bill found the appropriate playing partners.

In 2002 Bill Hancock retired as a lawyer and became a starter, the person who acts as a sort of traffic cop and gatekeeper on the first tee of a busy golf course. It is the starter who oversees that symbolic launching point to a day of golf and oversees, ultimately, who tees off and when.

When Hancock went to work at the public Ballyowen Golf Club in northwestern New Jersey, he thought he knew what he was getting into. He had been, after all, a lifelong golfer. He was in for a surprise. It turns out Bill's new trade requires the skills of several professions: tailor, seer, therapist, matchmaker. The starter or the caddie master, who can fill the same role at a private club, is very much like a concierge of golf and as such can hold the key to a great day.

Every golf course or golf club, whether it is public or private, has a fleet of professionals like Hancock waiting to be of assistance. They are a golfer's best friend. Far too many golfers pay little attention to these servants of the game, when there are clubhouse managers, locker room attendants, caddies, and starters who can demystify and resolve golf's various quandaries — on the course and, sometimes more important, off of it.

"Getting ready to play golf makes a lot of people nervous and befuddled," Hancock said. "There's a lot of running around and tension. I want people to be calm and enjoy the atmosphere. Sometimes, I'll stand by the first tee and sing to everyone on the practice green."

Ballyowen, a spectacular links-style layout with a Celtic theme, outfits its starters in kilts. Beside his starter's hut overlooking the dunes and wild fescue, Hancock sings a mean "Danny Boy."

"People stop, take in the setting, and maybe say to themselves, 'Hey, we're pretty lucky to be out here today,'" Hancock said.

Every golfer should find an extra hour or two someday just to stand on the first tee of a golf course. You will learn a lot about golfers, about recreational golf, and about yourself. It will improve your play and your perspective on our golfing pastime. You will see how your arrival at the golf course can set the tone for everything to follow, and it will probably alter how you approach that experience. After standing on the tee for a while, you should then wander around the grounds, from the pro shop to the caddie shack. That is where you will find the true oracles of information about that golf course and about recreational golf in general. As a golf writer it's been part of my job to take this tour of the grounds many times. Do you know what these golf lifers tell me over and over? That no one asks them any questions. No one seems to want to know the considerable number of things they know.

"We can help the golfers who come here with pretty much everything they need or want to know," said John Wesoloski, the longtime locker room attendant at the Ridgewood Country Club, the New Jersey setting for a PGA Tour event, regional competitions, and an active schedule of local membership golf, too. "We've seen it all. And you can see that people have a lot of questions. But most of them don't ask us. I don't know why."

It's likely that arriving golfers don't want to bother anyone. Or they feel embarrassed or inhibited by the setting. But the fact is that most people who work at a golf course do so because they like being around golf. Talking to them about their job or workplace gives them another opportunity to talk about golf, and by asking questions you are flattering them, acknowledging that they can help you.

Consider the starter, someone whom people often zoom past in their carts on the way to the first tee. The starter knows the course maintenance mowing schedule and so knows the speed of the greens that day. You might want to ask about that. The starter also knows where the rough is likely to be highest. Another good thing to know. The starter knows where the pins are placed. The starter can recommend what tees to play from. The starter knows how much water or rain the greens have received and can tell you if they're soft or hard.

Why in the world would anybody overlook someone like that? But people do it all the time.

"People should realize that we are all in this together," Hancock said. "The golfers and the people who work at the golf course, we all want you to play your best. That's good for everybody, good for the pace of play, good for everybody's mood, and good for business. People should know it's all of us together against the golf course. We'll do whatever it takes to help."

There are other key people at the familiar points of entry to the golfing experience. If you are a guest at a private club, for example, the first person you meet could be the locker room attendant, another pivotal friend in waiting. My first advice in maximizing this relationship is to be early.

"A lot of people don't arrive early enough for their tee time to enjoy all the benefits of a club," says Rob Bucci, the caddie master at the Ardsley Country Club in Westchester County outside New York City. "It's not a big deal, but we're here to take care of you. Come early; we'll make you comfortable and get you whatever you need. You can warm up and practice. If you rush in at the last minute, you're missing that chance."

When invited to play in an outing at a private club, a lot of people worry about breaking unspoken protocols.

"It is probably not a good idea to show up in denim jeans with your baseball cap on backwards," said Bucci, who is a past president of the national Caddie Masters Association. "Cell phone use is something that should be avoided. But usually it's not anything that hard or fancy. If somebody is really worried about it, the best thing they can do is go to the caddie master and say, 'Hey, I've never done this before.'

"That's when we're at our best."

Willie Logan, the locker room attendant at the Colorado Golf Club, once told me he thought the locker room existed for more than the obvious — a restroom, showers, and a place to change clothes and shoes. It was Logan's belief that the atmosphere of the locker room — convivial and comfy, where every need is within arm's reach — existed to shed any aura of anxiety about the approaching golf round. The locker room is a place of attitude adjustment. You walk through the door and leave behind the rest of the world. In the locker room you have an adult version of a child's playroom — televisions tuned to sports, card tables, and friends talking about nothing more consequential than something called a birdie or a bogey. The place delivers a clear message: We are here to play a game. Now go out there and have fun.

But what about the club etiquette in this sanctuary-like environment? Well, it's not quite like entering a secret society even if people like to imagine that it is. Harry Potter had it much harder at Hogwarts. There are only a very few don'ts and just a few places to be careful. For example, don't change your shoes in the parking lot. That's a no-no. Carry your golf shoes in a bag and change them in the locker room. If you have bought a travel bag for checking your golf clubs on the airlines, it likely came with a shoe bag that unzips from the travel case. That's a good shoe bag for visiting the country club.

Any other Emily Post–like etiquette is fairly straightforward. Clubs sometimes have specific rules for the grill or the bar — such as prohibiting hats and caps. It's probably a good idea to remove your hat regardless, unless you are on the golf course or in the locker room.

In general, during your visit, wear your best golf duds. The bar on clothing is not very high — this is golf, not fashion week in Milan. Clean is good; avoid tattered.

Refrain from smoking except where it is permitted.

Keep your voice down.

Don't be showy. Don't talk about all the other clubs you have visited.

Smile, say "please" and "thank you" often, and look people in the eye. In other words, be polite; that always goes a long way.

It's not that big a deal. We are no longer living in 1965 when there really was a country club society apart from the rest of us. These days, the vast majority of clubs are looking for members. You are welcome.

Besides, trust me, at most clubs the staff grouses about the members, not the guests. The guests are a happy interlude. But as a guest, you have to deal with the matter of tipping. This unwritten social contract rewarding good service vexes many people at public and private courses alike. It can be a little hard to grasp, especially since the tipping predicament can begin the moment you pull into the parking lot and those kids in carts come chasing after your car. One kid fetches the clubs out of your trunk, then hands them to another kid 2 feet away. So do you tip both of them? And how much? The whole thing sometimes can make a visitor uneasy. It's not just the cart boys; there is the caddie master, the starter, the locker room attendant, the beverage cart person, the caddie, then the cart boys again. Maybe that is why people don't ask for help at the golf course — they are afraid it will lead to a tip.

What to do?

The first thing you should do in this setting is relax. So many golfers and so many guests come through private clubs and exclusive resorts every day that there is nothing you can do, or not do, that will leave a lasting impression. Unless you deposit your cart in a pond so that it has to be towed out (I've seen that), or unless you nearly bean the club president's wife with an errant shot as she sits on the club patio (I've done that), there isn't much the staff hasn't already seen.

So don't fret. Smile and act as if you're happy to be there, which you should be. That's step one. And, know that you don't have to tip someone just because he or she answers a question. But you will probably have to tip a certain number of staff members. Who, and how much?

Let's start with the realization that all tipping is subjective and personal. There are no hard-and-fast rules, and it's based on the quality of the service. But I know what you're thinking: You don't want to be a poor guest. You don't want to be called cheap or do anything that might reflect on your host, the club member. So here's what you do, based on numerous conversations with employees in each job.

Though you might be tempted to park in the lower, employees lot to avoid the cart boys or girls, don't run from them. They are just trying to help. Give them $2 or $3 per bag. You'll be off to a good start. If you feel comfortable doing so, it might be a good idea to call your host before the outing and ask about the club's tipping policies. You never know; there could be a no-tipping policy. It happens. Anyway, your host can eliminate a lot of indecision and fill you in on any other rules. There might be a no-shorts rule or, more commonly, no cargo shorts.

OK, but what if you haven't had the chance to talk to your host? In that case, when you get to the locker room, greet the locker room attendant and be up front about any questions you have. Don't just wander around clueless. Ask for help. "If people ask, we go out of our way to help," said Wesoloski, the Ridgewood locker room attendant. "It's understandable that some people who play at public courses might not be used to our routines. But those routines are not anything secret. We can get you a locker, we can tell you where things are. We can show you where you need to go to hit balls and introduce you to everyone you need to know."

If the locker room attendant cleans and shines your shoes for you, tip the attendant $5 to $10 per pair of shoes. A bigger tip might be appropriate if the attendant did anything else special for you — got you a Band-Aid and ointment for a blister or a drink after your round. If there is a caddie master, you might want to inquire about the base caddie rates, or anything else that might be expected of you. Again, your host might have already taken care of that, but you could offer to pay for the caddies or at least their tips. If you want a seasoned, high-quality caddie, sometimes it is worth it to tip the caddie master about 20 percent of the base caddie rate for the extra consideration.

Along the same lines, if you find yourself at a busy resort that has a starter and you want a preferred tee time, or the starter did some juggling to fit you in, a group of four golfers might want to tip the starter $50 or more should the starter have gone out of his or her way. It's not required, and it's not a bribe, just a gesture of thanks. While on the golf course, the beverage cart person should receive a tip not unlike the tip you would give a bartender. A soda and snacks cost $3? Hand over at least a buck. Bigger order? Bigger tip.

Caddies often receive a tip equal to 50 percent of the base caddie rate, though tips vary greatly from club to club and region to region. It can be as little as $10 in some quarters and $75 in others. It's a good idea to ask your host or others you might be playing with. Don't be embarrassed; just ask. If you have a forecaddie who is assisting your cart-riding group but not carrying the clubs, figure a tip of about $20 per person. When you come off the course, there might be some more cart attendants offering to clean your golf clubs as they take them off the cart. Again, about $2 or $3 per bag. You might want to offer to take care of this tip for your host as well.

So there, what did that come to? Maybe about $50 to $60, or roughly the same cost as the weekend golf rate with a cart at a public course. Depending on where you live, $50 or $60 might be more than you usually spend. But you received a lot of attention you wouldn't normally get, and that's the point. Enjoy the service and enjoy an atmosphere where everyone is simply trying to help you have a good day of golf. Enjoy the attention; everyone likes to be pampered.

Sometimes that attention includes the services of a caddie. This is a real treat that might save you five to ten strokes per round. Unfortunately, some people are uncomfortable having another set of eyes watching their every golf move.

"A lot of people, especially New York municipal course players, are intimidated by having to play with a caddie," said John Amoruso, the caddie master at Elmwood Country Club in White Plains. "They think the caddie is there to judge them, like they go somewhere later and laugh at them. The caddie doesn't care. Do you know how much bad golf that caddie has seen? He's seen people hit it backward off the first tee over and over. He's caught balls hit sideways at him.

"The caddie only wants to help you. Because if you relax, it's a better day for him, too. He gives you advice on how to play the course and how to approach things. It's the caddie's constant affirmation on how to play a hole that relieves the tension of playing somewhere unfamiliar. People should enjoy having a friend and part-time psychologist out there with them."

A good caddie, and even a bad one, which is rarer, can turn any golf round into a stroll in the park. Literally. How great is it to hit a shot, hand someone your club, and walk through the verdant landscape? This agreeable way to play the game has been around since the sixteenth century. When Mary Queen of Scots played golf in Scotland back then, she made sure her sons caddied for her. It's said they kept her from losing her head on the links, something they had more trouble doing years later.

At any rate, a good caddie quickly sizes up your game and can advise you how to get around the golf course, a layout with which you may not be familiar. A good caddie can read the greens for you, invaluable assistance when playing a new course. Most of all, it is reassuring to have another informed opinion on where to aim, what club to hit, and what club not to hit. In this way, a good caddie clears your head of the internal distracting chatter in the sometimes tense moments before a shot is struck. At its best, playing with a caddie can be a four- or five-hour symbiotic experience that relies heavily on the caddie's ability to keep the golfer upbeat.

I remember playing in Florida one day when every approach shot to every green seemed to fade right and end up 20 to 25 feet from the pin. I was reaching greens in regulation; I just couldn't hit my irons perfectly straight. It was starting to bug me, and I kept focusing on the negative part of those outcomes. When it happened for maybe the eighth time in twelve holes, I complained: "Another one to the right. Why does that keep happening?"

My caddie, a young man who caddied by day and waited tables at an Outback restaurant at night, walked past me and said: "Yeah, it must suck having all those birdie putts." That put me in my place. He was right; so it wasn't perfect, but I was still compiling a good score. I spent the next six holes looking at the glass as half full and had a great day. I think I even started hitting it straighter.

Average golfers could get a lot more out of the player-caddie relationship if they saw the golf round through the caddie's eyes. Theirs is a tough job. A couple of years ago, I caddied for the LPGA star Brittany Lincicome for one day of an official tournament in New Jersey. That was nerve-racking.

I remember one early hole. I was especially jumpy. It wasn't about choosing the right club to hit or helping read a worrisome birdie putt. No, I was certain I had lost two of Lincicome's club head covers. Oh, and when she asked for the golf ball she had just handed me to clean, at that particular moment I could not find that, either.

As I said, caddying is hard, especially when it is for a top pro who

a. hits the ball 285 yards (hard to see that far);
b. hits shots precise yardages and requires accurate pre-shot distance calculations (so much math);
c. putts perfectly straight but wants a seasoned eye to point the safe path through every green's hills and swales (who am I, Sacajawea?);
d. expects you not to lose her stuff, most especially her golf ball seconds after marking it and placing it in your palm (caddie jumpsuits have too many pockets).

In all seriousness, it's a demanding assignment. First of all, a tour pro's bag is heavy, laden with balls, clubs, towels, notebooks, tools, rain clothes, and snacks. It is wide and bulky to make room for sponsors' logos. It might weigh thirty-five pounds. For the first few holes, that weighs on your shoulder. By the tenth, it weighs on your back because your shoulder is numb. Making things much worse is that the golfers walk fast — they are young and in shape — and you are usually expected to get to the ball, wherever it is, about when they do. You must do this even though you might have to first chase after a divot, grab it and replace it, then clean the club the player just hit with a wet towel, put the club away, and lift the bag to your shoulder, again.

The routine never changes: Comment on shot ("Nice ball"), get divot, clean club, chase everyone down the fairway. When you catch up at the ball, you have to pull out the course's yardage book, which has annotations, markings, and drawings that resemble Egyptian hieroglyphics. In a matter of seconds, you find a nearby sprinkler head or edge of a bunker, which, according to the book, is, let's say, 125 yards from the front of the green. You march off how many yards your player's ball is from this landmark. Let's say in this case it is 5 yards farther from the green.

Then you consult your pin-placement page, which shows where the hole has been placed on all eighteen greens. You find the appropriate green and see that the hole is 6 yards from the front of the green. Then you check the personal caddie notes you would have made two or three days earlier while walking the course with a range finder and see that shots to this particular green will play 3 yards farther because the green is elevated above the fairway. At this point, you might also factor in wind (no charts for that, just an experienced estimate).

Anyway, at that point, you declare to the player: "It's 136 yards playing uphill, so the number is 139." And don't forget that number.

On one hole when I was caddying for Lincicome, I gave her a yardage figure, and then a few minutes passed as she waited for her playing partners to hit their shots. When it was her turn, she stood over her ball, then hesitated.

"What was the number again, Bill?" she said.

I had completely forgotten — there had been so many numbers already. And did I tell you my shoulder was numb?

Lincicome, who could not be more polite and pleasant, waited as the number was calculated again. Later, she explained what makes a caddie-player relationship work — in any setting, on any golf course.

"The relationship becomes personal on some level," she said. "You're out there five hours a day and a lot happens, some of it bad. The game of golf can make you feel lonely and you need a friend. When I've just made an 8 on a hole and I need someone to find a way to change the mood so I calm down, that's a good caddie."

I did make it all the way through my round with Lincicome and she played well, even making a 40-foot birdie putt as I held the flag on the eighteenth hole. I was happier still when I realized I had ibuprofen in my pocket to wash down at the nineteenth hole. As for that early mishap, I did soon find the head covers, which had slipped to the bottom of the bag. And after a few seconds of fumbling in my pockets, I even discovered Brittany's ball. Well, I'm still not certain it was the one she gave me, but it was round and it was white. I handed it over and I said something like "Knock it in."

I felt like a good caddie when she did.

But my caddying experience taught me some other things because I got to hang around for a few days with all the real caddies, including many who continued to carry clubs for recreational golfers. That was educational. Some of them said they had caddied more than 7,000 rounds in their lives. And those were the young ones with good memories; the real vets gave up counting a long time ago.

Caddies, you may have heard, can be a salty, entertaining, and opinionated crew. I asked for their chief suggestions on how players can make them happy and eager to help throughout the day. OK, I never asked; they just told me. Here are some highlights:

Take all the extra stuff in your bag out and leave it in the trunk of your car. We all get used to riding in golf carts when it doesn't matter if there are three windbreakers, an extra pair of shoes, a metal swing-training aid, and forty-five balls in the bag. If you're about to play at a club with caddies, however, remove everything superfluous. That probably includes half the balls in your bag.

It's part of the caddie's job to give you yardage to the hole, but don't be too picky. Nothing is worse, my new caddie buddies said, than some guy who is lying 6 and hasn't made a single consistent swing all day insisting on knowing whether his seventh shot is going to be 103 yards or 100 yards to the middle of the green. Interestingly, they said that the better players often just want general yardage because they know the shot's shape and trajectory will determine what they hit, not necessarily the exact yardage.

Don't load up on fancy clubs. Remember, only fourteen, but in reality most caddies think average golfers carry too many clubs, anyway. One caddie suggested that golfers with a handicap of 20 or higher should be prohibited from carrying more than ten clubs because they would become better, faster, if they learned to hit a variety of shots with fewer clubs. They might also learn to be consistent with the clubs they had.

If you are in a bunker and fail to get your shot out of the bunker but hit it 25 feet to another portion of the bunker, don't start trudging across the sand, walking across the whole bunker to your ball for your next shot. Instead, step out onto the grass and walk around as close as you can to your ball and reenter the bunker. Remember, the caddie has to rake all of your footprints after your two, or three, shots.

In the end, playing with a good caddie can make golf a team game, and that is something to be prized. It helps the golf partnership experience blossom, and it's something to relish. It also makes a long, hard golf course less intimidating. We will tackle it together, shot by shot. This can, of course, also be done in team format matches with your friends. But the caddie connection is different still, because only one person continues to hit the shots. There is a connection nonetheless. The caddie is the only person recognized in the Rules of Golf who can legally provide advice of any kind to a player (if the caddie breaches a Rule, the player can also be penalized).

Arnold Palmer said that all golfers have an inner caddie, but it helps to have a tangible one standing alongside for affirmation. In the book *Think Like a Caddie, Play Like a Pro*, which was produced by the Professional Caddies Association, Jack Nicklaus talks about the most important 6 inches in golf — the space from the left ear to the right ear. Caddies hand us clubs and lug the bag, but they help golfers control those important 6 inches. In the same book, Ben Crenshaw writes about how having a caddie means never having to walk to a poor shot alone. He's right. It's already a lonesome feeling out there, but it can get better with another voice to lighten the mood or rechannel your focus.

Perhaps no golfer needed more help with his focus than Ben Crenshaw at the 1995 Masters tournament. Crenshaw grew up in Texas and learned the game from the iconic teacher Harvey Penick, who died the Sunday before the tournament was to begin. Crenshaw, the 1984 Masters winner, was already at Augusta National practicing when he heard the news of his beloved mentor's passing. Still, he remained for a practice round the next day but played very poorly.

At Augusta, Crenshaw had always used the same caddie, Carl "Skillet" Jackson, and during that 1995 practice round, Jackson spotted a flaw in Crenshaw's swing. In its most basic form, Crenshaw was standing too far from the ball. Crenshaw made the adjustment on the range after his practice round and immediately started striking the ball more crisply. Then he flew back to Texas to be a pallbearer for his mentor.

When Crenshaw returned and the tournament began, he was playing better, but he did so with a heavy heart. Harder still, every few minutes a few well-meaning spectators would offer Crenshaw their condolences.

"Ben was carrying a lot of weight that week," Jackson said. "I was carrying the bag but I had to help him carry some of the other stuff. And after all the conversation from the galleries — with Ben thanking people left and right — I had to get him refocused on the shot at hand. We understood the situation.

"But Mr. Penick's number one piece of advice was always 'Take dead aim.' Ben had to remember that too."

And so Crenshaw did, going seventy-two holes without a three-putt to win his second green jacket. When the final putt fell, he buried his face in the chest of the taller Jackson and wept. The scene — an Augusta black man, one of nine children in a single-parent home whose first golf job paid 75 cents a day, embracing the son of an upper-middle-class Texas country club family — is one of the most famous pictures in sports history.

Nicklaus had a longtime caddie relationship as well. Beginning in 1963, Angelo Argea, a former Las Vegas cabdriver who sported a full, wiry shock of silver hair, toted his bag.

"We had a sometimes indefinable connection," Nicklaus said of Argea, who remained Nicklaus's caddie for nearly twenty years.

The duo became a fixture in televised golf, the great Golden Bear who was on his way to becoming the best golfer in the world, and the tall, dark caddie with the big hair.

"Those were great times and he gave me what I needed," Nicklaus said. "He wasn't the type of caddie that talked me out of shots or gave me a lot of swing advice, but especially at that time I wasn't a player who needed that. There is more than one way to be a great caddie, but all good players need a caddie's help in some way."

So do lesser players, perhaps even more so.

Playing the Carnoustie Golf Links in Scotland years ago, I hit a dreadful shot into some heather and left myself about 180 yards from the green. Embarrassed and frustrated, I didn't say a word as I trudged to the ball. Then I turned to my caddie: "What do you think? Can I get there with a 4-iron?"

Looking at my lie in the thick stuff, my caddie answered: "Eventually."

Of course, I laughed. And came to my senses. I hit a wedge back to the fairway and moved on without any real incident. I actually played pretty well thereafter, snickering every so often as I recalled our earlier conversation. Buying my caddie a pint a few hours later, I toasted him with one memorable word: "Eventually."

There is a last best friend eager to help at the golf course, and the practice range, and golfers everywhere should raise a glass to that person as well. If this is a chapter about the oracles of golf information who plainly can lead us out of the woods, there are no more important prophets, psychics, mystics, and diviners than the nearly 30,000 golf teaching pros. A certified PGA professional has taken courses not only in swing instruction but in the business of golf, club fitting, managing oneself on the golf course, and another four or five subjects. A good golf pro can teach you to putt, chip, pitch, shape the ball left and right, get out of the sand, and get out of the rough. The golf pro can teach you how to practice, how to warm up for a round, and how to end one: Take your hat off and shake hands.

Many people play golf all their lives and never take a lesson or ask the help of a PGA pro. Many of them are even good golfers, but frankly, I'm not sure why they would torture themselves like that. To me, playing golf sometimes feels like living in a country where the people speak a language that is an incomprehensible jumble of symbols. There's not even an alphabet. So all the road signs, menus, and conversations are indecipherable. The golfer keeps trying to figure out this strange language but can't.

Taking a good golf lesson makes me feel as if someone has finally given me a dictionary or legend to the symbols of this strange other world. The PGA pro has the answers, and all you need to do is ask for his or her help. But many people avoid the teaching pro, as if the pro might ruin their golf game. Ruin it? The average score of the average golfer has not changed in forty years. It still hovers around 100 for eighteen holes. How much worse could we all get?

Other people feel like they're not good enough to take a lesson. This is the craziest notion of all.

"Simple fundamentals of grip, stance, and alignment could make all the difference in the world," said Joe Hallett, the former director of the PGA Center for Golf Learning and Performance. "Some people are doing the basics so wrong, it's like they're playing blindfolded. We can take off the blindfold and you would be surprised how much easier they suddenly find golf."

Other golfers feel as if they don't play enough golf to take a lesson. Or don't have time to practice, so what's the point? I've felt this way myself from time to time, but I've come to look at it this way: Even if you play just ten times a year, which means you spend on average at least $300 and maybe as much as $700 a year on golf rounds, would you not pay another $50 to cut five to seven strokes off your score in each of those ten rounds? If you shoot about 100, that's entirely doable after one lesson.

OK, so lessons, or at least a few lessons, are important but only as important as what you get out of them. Even if it's one hour once a year, which might be enough for many veteran players, you should make the most of it. I have consulted some of the most respected teachers in the world about how to do this. Here is what they had to say:

Tip No. 1: Be on time. Better yet, be early.

This is the second time punctuality has come up but it's important. If you don't arrive early enough to warm up, relax, and clear your head, you probably won't learn as much. "People show up tight, stressed, and in a hurry," Jim Suttie, ranked sixteenth on the *Golf Digest* list of top American golf instructors, said. "Golf is recreation, and a golf lesson should be fun. Take the time to swing the club for ten or fifteen minutes, to loosen up and calm down." Warming up also allows you to start swinging as you normally do — you know, launching balls left and right or dribbled along the ground. Hey, that's why you're taking a lesson.

Tip No. 2: Don't tell the instructor what's wrong with your swing.

This was mentioned several times by the pros. Golfers show up and say, "I need a quicker transition." Or "My left arm is stuck inside." These are all things analysts say during televised golf broadcasts, and unless you frequently play on TV, they probably are not talking about you. "A good instructor will understand what's going on with your swing after you've hit three balls," Laird Small (number 32, *Golf Digest*) said. "There is other info that might be more useful for the instructor at the beginning of the lesson." Which leads to . . .

Tip No. 3: Do tell the pro what's been going wrong.

There is a big difference between telling the instructor what's wrong with your swing and explaining what has been happening to your golf ball. "It is helpful to hear that most shots have been going right to left or just way right," Don Hurter (number 42) said.

Mike Bender (number 9) added: "You should arm the instructor with a little description of your typical game. Describe what's wrong like you would in a doctor's office."

Tip No. 4: Listen.

"People are used to talking," said Suttie, who teaches at the Cog Hill Golf and Country Club outside Chicago. "But they often aren't very good listeners. A good teacher will take in everything you've said and make up a plan for helping you. But you have to hear the message, understand the solution, and understand why it will work." If you don't understand, the pros said, don't be afraid to ask questions. They have lots of ways of explaining the same thing.

Tip No. 5: Be open to new ideas.

"Students shouldn't get defensive," said Dana Rader, number 46 and one of five women on the *Golf Digest* list. "The teacher might change a grip, and yes, it won't feel normal. But I tell my students the reasons why a new grip might help. And I ask them to trust me for three or five swings. Give it a try with an open mind."

Tip No. 6: Be honest with your teacher.

How much time do you have to practice? If the answer is never, the instructor may give you some drills you can do in front of a mirror at home or during a break at work. And if you are a terrible putter, say so. Don't say you're OK because you think you can fix it yourself. If you haven't fixed it by now, you probably need the help.

Tip No. 7: Do your homework before selecting a teacher.

"If you had a serious illness, you would do research on whom to see, but people will take a golf lesson from anybody who says he's a pro," said Bender, whose golf academy is in Lake Mary, Florida. "Find out a little about your instructor and his teaching methods and consider whether it would be a good fit for you. You could meet with or call the teacher beforehand."

Sometimes the first lesson is like making a new friend or a new business partner. "You do need a connection with your teacher," said Rader, whose golf school is in Charlotte, North Carolina. "The teacher needs to make the student comfortable. And the teacher needs to adjust to the student; it's certainly not the other way around. Students should make sure that is the kind of teacher they are getting."

Tip No. 8: Finally, set reachable goals, because one lesson isn't meant to overhaul your game, just improve it.

"People sometimes expect miracles," said Don Hurter, the head professional at Colorado's Castle Pines Golf Club. "We usually have to teach in small pieces that add up to a lot. For example, lots of people want to hit the ball farther, and a lot of them slice their shots, too. We usually can fix a slice, and if I get you drawing the ball into the center of the fairway, it is going farther. One thing at a time."

Again, if you think you don't need the help, keep in the mind that the greatest golfers in the world all have teachers.

Phil Mickelson, who has one of the best and most imaginative short games in golf history, has a special short-game coach, the noted short-game guru Dave Pelz. And it wasn't as if Pelz sought the job.

"When Phil called me," Pelz said, "my first reaction was to ask him: 'Phil, what in the world do you need me for?'"

Mickelson had an answer.

"I want to be a quarter of a shot better per round in the majors," he said.

In other words, one stroke better by the end of the tournament. Mickelson first contacted Pelz in 2003 when he had not won a major but had come in second often. He won his first Masters, by one stroke, one year later.

This is a different world from what the recreational golfer seeks from a trip to the local PGA pro. Or is it?

"I don't know if it is all that different," Mickelson told me years ago. "Yes, I'm working on things at a very finite level and with a lot on the line. But I am trying to improve just one small thing just a little bit because it can have a big impact, like one stroke per four rounds.

"But the average golfer could also be working on one small thing, like getting out of every bunker in one stroke. You know, he never again wants to leave a ball in the sand. That can have a huge impact, not only because it might immediately save three shots a round but because that golfer now doesn't fear sand shots. That then affects how he or she hits all future approach shots to greens. Maybe there is the confidence to go for some pins now. And what goes with that? A less tense swing because there's less fear if the shot is short of right and ends up in a bunker. So there's another few strokes. And if it does end up in the bunker, maybe with new knowledge on how to play the shot, there develops more of an effort to get the ball close to the hole instead of just getting it out. That leads to one- or two-putts instead of three-putts.

"So is one good bunker lesson a small thing? No way, not at all. It's a big thing just like my short-game lessons are for me."

In 2010, when Tiger Woods tried coaching himself, he had the worst results of his professional career. Yes, there were extenuating circumstances — to say the least — but his swing was also a total mess.

And Woods had no shortage of video analysis to view as a self-coach, not to mention an encyclopedic knowledge of the golf swing. Still, he couldn't fix himself.

Imagine how out of whack the average player can get without much, if any, video to analyze and with little expert knowledge of the dynamics of the swing.

Laird Small, director of the Pebble Beach Golf Academy in California, says he prefers to learn a student's overall golf goals before a lesson. "I like it when someone says, 'I am an 18 handicap and I'm not trying to be a 10 handicap, but right now I'm playing like I'm a 25 handicap and I should be better than that,'" said Small, the 2003 PGA Teacher of the Year. "Somebody else might say they are an 18 who wants to get to be a 12 handicap. The prescriptions for fixing those two situations are completely different. But I can help in both situations if I understand the goals ahead of time."

Suttie has found better results sometimes by moving the golf lesson from the range to the golf course where he conducts a playing lesson. "On the range, hitting balls over and over, people often perform better," Suttie said. "Sometimes you get a real read of their game watching them hit shots that count."

Don Hurter agreed. "You can learn a lot and help someone a lot thereafter by just playing five holes with them," he said.

Small suggested that students hit their favorite club for a teacher and also hit their least favorite club. "Sometimes the biggest flaw is revealed with the least favorite club," he said. "And that might be the one you want to go after."

Dana Rader recommends that golfers divulge any physical limitations they might have before the lesson. "Did you recently have knee surgery?" she says. "Do you have a back problem or anything else that might be limiting you?"

After talking with hundreds of pro teachers, I've come away with how much time and thought they have put into helping their students. I've spent countless hours with them and attended their national conventions. You wouldn't believe the arguments they can get into over the best way to cure an over-the-top swing move. First, they'll argue for an hour about whether it should even be called "over-the-top" be-cause some older teacher called the move a "slingshot maneuver" in 1912 and then it was called an "outside loop" in the 1950s. They will snatch smartphones from their pockets and start displaying and ana-lyzing all the golf swing videos they've saved and cataloged. They will argue about relevant historical swing theory precedents like a bunch of Constitutional lawyers — Bobby Jones versus Ernest Jones — and they will ruminate about whether you should look at the hole or the ball when putting. Don't get them started on ball position; you'll miss your morning tee time.

OK, so they are obsessed. But they are obsessed because golf is fasci-nating to them and making every golfer happier is their mission. They never argue about their own swings or their own golf games. It is as if they never get to play, which is sometimes closer to the truth than it would seem. So they obsess about making us better instead. What did the starter Bill Hancock say? We're all in this together.

What does all this mean? We as everyday golfers should pay a lot more attention to the golf professionals who want to help us. Because they have invested a lot of time in how to best offer that help.

Golf pros, locker room attendants, caddies, and starters — they are there for you. You are not alone out there. This is not a minor thing. There is no game that can make you feel friendless and aban-doned faster and more completely than golf. But you do not walk — or ride — alone. Know there is help and know where it is. You won't be sorry.

The next time you head to the first tee, remember that whatever happens — even if you split your pants — somebody has your back (side).

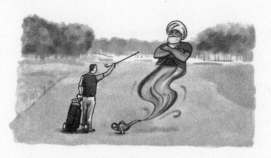

6

If You Had One Wish . . .

The reason the pro tells you to keep your head down
is so you can't see him laughing.

PHYLLIS DILLER

PLAYING A SOLITARY round on a quiet weekday evening at my home course, I searched for an errant shot in the woods and came upon a stray golf ball.

The ball had a smudge of dirt on it. I tried to rub it off, but the smudge wouldn't budge. I rubbed harder and harder, and suddenly — in a puff of white smoke — there appeared a genie.

With an Augusta National towel wrapped around his head and a golf ball earring dangling on one side, he stood before me, his arms folded ominously on top of an ample belly. He roared, "I am the golf genie, and I am here to grant you one wish."

Not that this happens every day, but I wondered, "Isn't it supposed to be three wishes?"

The genie scowled.

"Didn't anyone ever tell you golf is unfair?"

"Yeah."

"Well, so is the golf genie. You get one wish for anything you want in your golf game."

I looked around. We were alone.

"Anything?" I said, my mind racing. "Like Phil Mickelson's short game? His long game? His putting? His bank account?"

The genie frowned.

"No, no, no, and what's the matter with you?" he said. "Look, you can have just one shot, like a drive, a pitch, a chip, or a putt. But forevermore, as long as you play golf, you will execute that shot perfectly.

"In other words, your driver will go 300 yards and straight every time. Or every putt from less than 6 feet will always go in the hole. Every pitching wedge will land within 6 feet of the flagstick, or every bunker shot will settle within 2 feet of the hole."

The genie laughed devilishly.

"So, my wayward golfing friend, what's your pleasure?"

I couldn't organize my thoughts. Who wouldn't want to make every short putt forever? Goodbye to those humiliating yips.

Then again, 300-yard drives every time? Hello, testosterone rush — like taking steroids without having to appear at a congressional hearing.

The genie was talking again.

"Now, a few ground rules. I don't do aces — no holes in one every time on a par 3. You can't ask for all your irons to go the perfect distance, just one. Work with me."

The genie cocked an eyebrow as he eyed me up and down.

"You look like somebody who can't hit a pitching wedge straight to save your life," he said. "How about I fix that for you?"

That sounded so puny. I was choosing a shot for all golfing eternity. I wanted a shot that would make my golfing buddies cry out and my golf opponents simply cry.

A precise pitching wedge? Oooh, I'm scared.

"OK, look, how about I fix your short game around the green?" the genie suggested.

Now I was frowning.

"Are you a genie or Dave Pelz?" I said.

The genie was getting exasperated. He started spitting out possible wishes for me:

"Every ball you hit in the trees will automatically bounce out. . . ."

"Tuck your right elbow perfectly every time in the backswing. . . ."

"No shot ever rolls into a divot. . . ."

"Hit it low in the wind every time. . . ."

"If someone near you on the golf course is using a cell phone, his pants will automatically fall down around his ankles. . . ."

I just kept shaking my head and saying, "No."

"This is why it takes five hours to play eighteen holes," the genie said. "No one can make up their mind out here."

Let me ask you: What would you choose?

I've asked many of my friends. Some are wise guys. One guy said he would ask to be invisible for at least five seconds after every tee shot so he could grab his ball and throw it farther down the fairway. I reminded him that assumes he could find his tee shot.

Another friend said he would want every one of his shots to go 2 yards farther than every shot struck by his father-in-law. "I'll be perfectly happy with a 100-yard drive if his was only 98 yards," my friend said with delight in his eyes. "My father-in-law would go nuts. He'd be chucking clubs all over the place."

Golf does indeed make strange bedfellows.

Another friend wanted the psychic ability to bend the shots of his opponents. He wanted to be able to stare at a ball and make it slice into the woods or plop in a pond. "I don't want to play any better; I just want others to play as badly as I do," he said.

Whoa. Have I ever mentioned that golf makes people crazy?

But back here in the world of relatively sane golfers, the genie's query is intriguing. We all have things we would like to perfect in our golf games, but this is a different question: What is the one shot you wish you had forever? It's almost like a biblical parable or an allegory that lays bare the real meaning of golf, or life.

Either that or it's a way to win more $2 Nassaus.

At any rate, most people seem to believe the answer has to vary from player to player. Most of us, and this goes for professional players as well, are usually better at hitting our irons or our woods. Almost everyone has a few clubs that are a little more dependable and a little less erratic than the other clubs. This is partly true because the iron swing and wood swing are inescapably different. Some instructors preach that it's all one swing and always the same. They say the only thing that changes is the ball position. But even they usually temper those statements by admitting that what also changes is the club's angle of attack.

In physics, this might make sense. In golf, it comes down to this: The one thing most golfers come to realize is that altering the angle of attack changes the swing in a major way. Sweeping a ball off a tee or a tight fairway with a wood is far different from contacting the ball first and then the turf with the steeply descending arc of an iron. The fact is, most of us are better with the shorter clubs or the longer ones.

So is the ultimate golf wish question as simple as fixing your weaker element? Wait a minute, this is golf. Nothing can be that simple.

I wanted to know what golf teachers would say. They are the people who have assessed amateur golf swings by the thousands, sometimes across three or four decades. I contacted a dozen from the list of *Golf Digest*'s top fifty American golf instructors, many of them the biggest names in golf teaching or coaching.

I put the genie conversation to them, which was a scenario that strangely didn't even faze them (veteran golf types will apparently believe anything). They had a lot of opinions.

Jim Hardy, the 2007 PGA Teacher of the Year and consistently ranked among the *Golf Digest* top ten teachers, said this:

"The most valuable shot in golf is the tee shot. Because most players are not just missing the fairway off the tee, they are barely keeping the ball on the planet. If someone could wish for one shot, it would be a straight, true tee shot."

Of course, Hardy had an odd way to accomplish this without a genie.

"Most players should take their driver outside right now, lay it down on their driveway, get in the car, and run it over five or six times until it's smashed completely," he said. "Then they would have to tee off with their 3-wood. And if after four months they have consistently kept the ball in play off the tee with the 3-wood, then they could consider buying another driver.

"But right now, the driver is killing most recreational players. That's their biggest problem by far."

Hardy had allies. Randy Smith, a top teacher from Dallas, said that inconsistent play off the tee made it impossible for regular players to score well.

"It's not so much distance, unless they're playing from tees they shouldn't be playing from," Smith said. "The bigger problem is hitting it in the rough or in the trees or over to the other hole. If you can teach someone to hit it straight off the tee, golf becomes a completely different game.

"There is nothing better for your golf game than to be calmly strolling off the tee, walking straight for a ball that you can see. It is so much harder trudging off to look for some ball buried in the rough or in some God-knows-where section near the out-of-bounds. When that happens, you walk off the tee knowing that at best you're going to have to hit some hybrid over a tree or some other miracle shot. You should probably chip back to the fairway, but even that is mildly demoralizing. Psychologically, you're already a mess.

"But if you put the ball plainly in view off the tee, everything changes. And it affects the likelihood of the next shot succeeding, too."

When I called Jim Flick, Jack Nicklaus's longtime teacher and another perennial top five pick in teacher rankings, and told him about my genie wish dilemma, he sounded as if he had met my genie.

"Oh, tell him you'll take the perfect driver every time," Flick said. "What a boost that would be. Who wouldn't want to start off every par 4 or par 5 with a perfect shot? And you probably would hit the next shot well because you're confident."

But from the beginning, I thought the other obvious choice was to want a putter that never missed, say, from 6 feet and in. I wondered if there wouldn't be a strong backlash from those advocating the putter. Wasn't it Ben Crenshaw who once said that the key to any good tee shot was making a par or birdie putt on the previous hole?

And I was right. The putter got a lot of votes.

Chuck Cook, another Texas-based top ten teacher: "If the average golfer could putt, he or she would automatically be five shots better. And that's for a 15 handicap. If you're a 25, then you'd be ten shots better."

John Elliott Jr. (number 38) agreed.

"Most people think they are pretty good putters because, let's face it, it looks easy," Elliott said. "No one wants to admit that they often — like three times a round — three-putt from 30 feet. But that is what we see. I'll take my students out and watch them in a little game of standard putting distances. The results are not pretty.

"So I would take the putter and as far as gaining confidence, I kind of think it might work the other way around. If players knew they were going to make a lot of putts, they would be more confident hitting their approach shots because they would know they don't have to hit it as close to the hole.

"Watch enough golf and you'll see that good putters are confident players."

Dean Reinmuth (number 48) had a similar take.

"If you made every 4- or 5-foot putt, you would be a very happy golfer," he said.

But Jim Hardy was still offering rebuttals (as I've said before, these guys don't agree much).

"Some people might choose the putter, but for the average player, that putt they miss for a 10 is not what's killing them," he said.

Just when I thought the discussion was restricted to a choice between the big dog and the flat stick, several teachers went to bat for the humble wedge.

That's what Mike LaBauve (number 31) voted for. "Hit your wedges close, and it will make your putting better — trust me," he said. "That's the primary scoring club, the wedge. It's not the driver and I can see the argument for the putter, but a good wedge player is almost always a good putter because he's not leaving himself many long putts.

"Plus, we all get in bad spots near the greens, and a great wedge player can make an important rescue shot."

Finally, I reached Butch Harmon, the top-ranked teacher on the list.

"Most people would choose the driver because they are enamored with distance," Harmon said. "Some other people might choose the putter because they have the yips or something. But what the average golfer should take is the wedge shot. That's the biggest stroke-saving shot.

"Great wedge play from 100 yards and in, man, that's like catching a genie in a bottle."

Whoa, this was getting freaky.

But now I was back to the puny wedge shot. I could not imagine that would be my pick for the perfectly struck golf shot throughout my golf eternity. It still felt deflating.

I decided to search for other experts, something like a golf analyst. No, not David Feherty, as entertaining as that might be (he'd probably recommend the ultimate ball retriever). I wanted someone who had broken golf down to a science. Golf is a game of numbers; perhaps a professor. Or a researcher. Or a professorial researcher!

And that's how I came upon Mark Broadie, a Columbia University graduate school professor of computational finance, avid golfer, and member of the United States Golf Association's handicap research team.

Broadie is one of those smart guys whom we regular, everyday golfers need. He is nearly a scratch golfer but highly curious about what makes some golfers proficient, others less so, and still others so bad they are downright desperate.

Broadie, who is in his mid-fifties, is a quiet and bookish-looking man. Thin and unimposing physically, he, like so many on the PGA and LPGA tours, is proof that successful golf is not linked to the size of one's biceps, height, or jacket size. So when I met Broadie in his Upper Manhattan home, I half expected him to deliver to me a tribute to the value of the short game.

We have, after all, heard this gospel all our lives: The key to low golf scores is a good short game. The vast majority of shots are struck from 100 yards and in; therefore, these are the most important shots in golf. It is accepted golf wisdom. But Broadie the golf stat geek is like Broadie the golfer — not someone to misjudge on the first tee.

In his Columbia office and at home, Broadie has a computer containing data from more than 80,000 — and counting — good, bad, and indifferent golf shots individually recorded by amateur golfers. Broadie, who uses mathematical models to evaluate the stock market, has spent more than seven years painstakingly collecting, storing, and analyzing shot data of amateurs and PGA Tour professionals in a computer program called Golfmetrics.

Broadie's research is the result of hundreds of hours of work by several associates, a professional computer programmer, and graduate students who assisted in technical aspects of the project. He wanted to assess the difference between a PGA Tour player's game and that of an amateur who shoots 75 or 85 or 100. The PGA Tour charts every shot by every player in every tournament, and Broadie obtained that research dating to 2003. He then had average golfers of all handicaps, from eight years old to seventy years old, start charting all their shots at various New York metropolitan-area golf courses, although most of this was done at his home course, the Pelham Country Club. The golfers shot from 65 to 155. Using Google Earth renderings of golf courses in the area and topographical booklets he made up, average golfers making notes during rounds on the golf course could record exactly where every shot went — in the fairway, in the rough, or out-of-bounds — and how far from the hole.

Broadie devised the Golfmetrics software application, and he and a few others entered the rounds in the computer program, documenting every putt, bunker shot, and other kind of shot — and the result. It took a few years, but the database has continued to grow.

The data allow Broadie to determine everything about how an average golfer plays. Not only can he determine how far the average low-, middle-, or high-handicap golfer hits a tee shot (the lower you score, the farther you tend to hit it), he can determine at what distance various golfers sink half their putts (8 feet for the PGA Tour pro, 6 feet for the player with a handicap from 0 to 9, 5 feet for those with a handicap from 10 to 19, 4 feet for someone with a handicap from 20 to 36).

Perhaps most valuable, he can analyze the value of each shot of a golfer's score.

And that is the genius and the most useful part of all of Broadie's work.

Because of his collection of 80,000-plus golf shots, Broadie has been able to assign a benchmark for performance from every spot on the golf course. To Broadie, the benchmark is the scratch golfer. Using his data, the professor has been able to determine, on average, how many strokes the scratch golfer would take to get the ball in the hole from almost anywhere on a golf course.

On a long par 4, it might take the scratch golfer, on average, about 4.6 strokes to finish the hole. From 80 yards away and in the sand, it takes about 2.9 strokes; from 160 yards away and on a par-3 tee, about 3.1 strokes — again, for the scratch golfer.

Once you have values for every shot, including putts and rescue shots, you can crunch the numbers for average golfers — easier to do if you're a professor of computational finance — and see where the most strokes are being lost compared to a top scratch player. In other words, how close in score were average golfers to the scratch golfer's average score of 3.1 on the 160-yard par 3? And how close were they to the scratch golfer's average score of 2.1 when putting from 28 feet?

The answer? Much closer while putting (2.4 strokes) than while teeing off on the par 3 (4.1 strokes).

Having the benchmark stroke averages allows Broadie to determine how and why 10, 20, 30, and 40 handicaps are most repetitively adding to their golf scores all around the golf course.

His findings would surprise most anyone linked to the golf community, where the short game rules — even a golf genie. For instance:

- In fact, it is the long game that proves to be the biggest factor when examining the difference in scores between pros and amateurs and even between low- and high-handicap amateurs. If, for example, a PGA Tour player were available to hit shots for an amateur from 100 yards and in, or available to hit all the shots leading to the 100-yard mark, Broadie says the amateur would benefit the most from having the PGA player hit the long shots, not the short ones.
- Having a pro putt for you would not accomplish as much as you might think. Broadie says the score for the average 16 handicap would be lowered by only 2.2 strokes if a PGA pro did all the putting. But if the PGA star hit all the shots outside 100 yards, the improvement would be 9.3 strokes.

- Despite the persistent belief that shorter hitters are more accurate off the tee than longer hitters, Broadie discovered the opposite: Longer hitters also tend to be straighter hitters. "Better players are more skilled overall," Broadie said. "They hit it farther and they have more consistent swings, so they're more accurate, too."

- Yes, as is often said, roughly 60 to 65 percent of all shots are struck within 100 yards of the hole. But Broadie noted that if you take out "gimme" putts of 2½ feet, the statistic has less meaning. Remove very short putts that are rarely missed, and shots from 100 yards or less account for only 45 to 50 percent of all shots. Eliminate putts from 3½ feet or less, and the figure drops to 41 to 47 percent.

Broadie, who is a 3 handicap, knows the heresy his research suggests. Not long ago, waiting for some groups to pass through Amen Corner at Augusta National, I ran into Dave Pelz and mentioned Broadie's stats to him. Pelz, who is a celebrated golf shot researcher himself, paused to look at me. Then his eyes widened and his face grew so red I thought I might have to shove him into Rae's Creek to cool him off.

"I can get the testimonies of thousands of players from my short-game schools who would say otherwise," Pelz, who is a large, imposing man, said in a half roar. "They improved by focusing on their short games."

When, in 2008, I wrote a newspaper story in *The New York Times* about Broadie — the first major publicity of his studies — readers who posted online comments were equally skeptical.

"Avoiding three-putts on any green is the key to scoring lower, I don't care what any Columbia egghead says," wrote one.

"Practice your chipping and your putting won't matter much," added another.

"I've learned to hit my 4-iron off every tee," wrote another. "It changed my life — no more searching for balls in the trees."

Wrote John from Thailand: "Golf is flog spelled backward."

While that might have temporarily leveled the debate, it did not make Broadie go away. His theories were presented to the World Congress of Golf, examined further in *Golf Magazine* and on the Golf Channel, and tossed back and forth in many a golf clubhouse, office lunchroom, and USGA symposium. No one could prove anything unquestionably — this is, after all, golf — but more important, no one could prove Broadie wrong.

Studying golf's intricacies is a mini industry in academia. Broadie is far from the only high-titled professor devoting hundreds of hours to golf research. There have been thousands of doctoral theses with golf as the central subject matter. But Broadie is out in front of the pack, and his USGA links have continued to give him some credibility in a contentious golf research community.

Aware of the pushback against his findings, Broadie tries to calm the furor by saying that he is not advocating that golfers spend less time practicing their short games, nor he is hoping we all abandon short-game clinics (half the golf instruction industry just exhaled a sigh of relief). He said, in fact, that his findings are not inconsistent with the accepted instruction doctrine that practicing the short game may be the easiest way to score lower.

"The data provide objective answers to where strokes are being lost, but the fact is if you've got two hours to practice, you probably won't start hitting the ball longer or straighter in that time period," Broadie said. "But you could probably get better at your putting or chipping in two hours of practice."

That doesn't change one of his basic discoveries — having Phil Mickelson, or any other top pro, hit tee shots for you would be more beneficial than having one of them putt for you. It is groundbreaking stuff. Now, admittedly, the sample used for Broadie's research is limited geographically, and women make up less than 20 percent of the group studied, a figure Broadie says he wishes were higher. But overall, he defends the sample as representative.

"I'm confident there is nothing atypical about Pelham Country Club golfers and others in the New York area I sampled," he said.

(For the record, I'm not taking sides. My short game is killing me. It happens right after my long game gets me in trouble.)

Golfmetrics, or something like it, will likely be a familiar part of the game in ten years. Just as early baseball statistical freethinkers like Bill James usurped traditional statistical measures like batting average, ERA, and RBI, Broadie and others have begun to remake how golfers will assess themselves.

At the Massachusetts Institute of Technology, researchers looked at every putt on thirty PGA Tour courses for five years beginning in 2003, which is about 2 million putts in total. They used their figures much as Broadie has. They know exactly how many strokes a PGA Tour pro usually needs to sink a 10-foot putt (1.63 strokes). This stat and others could become the benchmarks used to tell average golfers how well or poorly they putted on a given day. All the golfer would need to do is add up the distance of each of his or her initial putts that day and divide by the total number of putts. A table on the scorecard could tell the golfer how he or she did against a PGA Tour pro's average for those accumulated distances (with an adjustment for the severity and general contour makeup of the course).

Some days you might be four putts behind the pro, some days ten putts, but that would tell you how you did better than a simple total number of putts, which can often be more a reflection of how well you're chipping or hitting your approach shots. Similar tables could be added on the scorecard for shots all over the golf course.

In the meantime, there are some immediate practical uses. The PGA Tour and the USGA have spent a significant chunk of their vast resources applying mathematical formulas to the wealth of statistical data now available about every shot struck by a professional, and often by amateurs as well. Some of the results would not be surprising, but they help tell us about the average recreational game nonetheless. For example, at the end of how many rounds have you said, "If I just didn't take an 8 on the sixth hole, and then a 7 on the fifteenth hole, I would have had a pretty good day."

Do you believe that, or is it another misguided frequent golfer's lament?

It is basic truth, and even more true for a golfer with a high handicap. Someone who regularly shoots about 100 has four times as many blowup holes — with balls shanked into a pond or sliced into the deep woods — than someone who regularly shoots about 80.

"It sounds obvious but the really bad shots ruin more rounds than anyone suspects — it's probably the average golfer's biggest problem," said Jim Remy, the president of the PGA of America from 2010 to 2011. "Because if you hit a tee shot out-of-bounds, you're re-teeing and hitting three. But if you just mishit it a little and it scurries down the fairway 125 yards, at least you're only lying one and still have a shot at par.

"It's avoiding the shots that bring penalty strokes — in water hazards, out-of-bounds, lost balls — that is what matters. Those are the shots that destroy good rounds."

If you think about it, most of these big mistakes happen in the long game, not near the green. Yes, a three-putt is bad, but it's still only one more stroke than the average outcome. But when we're 190 yards from the green and trying some cockamamie cut shot with a hybrid because we saw Rickie Fowler do it on TV over the weekend, and it ends up in the school parking lot two holes away, well, that costs us a lot more than a stroke.

We have all heard the term *course management,* and most of us think it means laying up on long par 5s or occasionally hitting a 3-wood rather than a driver on a short par 4. It is actually far more involved than that, or should be. We should be adamant about our commitment to prevent the truly disastrous shots and constantly remind ourselves to hit a shot we have practiced often and can — most of the time — execute in a way that keeps the ball in the short grass.

Good course management can mean hitting a shot that greatly reduces the risk of causing a two-shot negative swing in your score — balls lost in the woods, dunked in a pond, or deposited in some family's garden birdbath out-of-bounds next to the green. This might mean hitting a club that may or may not get the ball all the way to the green but almost definitely won't result in one of those disastrous outcomes.

As Ben Hogan said: "Golf is not a game of good shots. It is a game of bad shots. It is a game of misses. The guy who misses the best is going to win."

And remember, the critical course management moment can also come after a miss. As golfers, we all seem to have the innate penchant to follow up one dreadful shot with an equally dreadful shot. Why?

Because we're frustrated and not thinking after the first miscue, and our subconscious is screaming that we've got to hit a wonderful shot to save face for the first blooper.

"You've really got to calm down after a bad shot and assess what's going on," said Don Hurter, one of *Golf Digest*'s top fifty instructors. "There's a good chance the hole can still be salvaged. Gather yourself, and really focus on what you're trying to do next so you can at least make double bogey. You might even make bogey.

"So, let's say you've hit it into the woods and are trying to punch out. Don't just grab a 4-iron and chop away. I see that all the time. And what often happens is that shot goes 40 yards farther than intended and rolls into a lake or into the woods on the other side of the fairway. Now you're still in trouble and even more upset. Plan your recovery with a clear head."

Of course, your head isn't very clear at that moment. You're worried about holding up your friends and you already feel silly. That doesn't mean you have to play silly. Just because, as nongolfers like to say, we are chasing a small white ball across the meadow until it is knocked into a seemingly smaller white hole, we don't have to lose our dignity.

Hold your head up, take deep breaths, and remember something motivational, like you could be at work instead, or be at the dentist's, or be a dentist at work.

In the end, remember that the golfer's pursuit is, in fact, incorporeal. The numbers of the game — and this chapter has a lot of them — are there to give the game a semblance of definition. They help us understand what we cannot understand — that we are trying to master that which cannot be mastered in the hope of mastering something greater within.

For whom are we chasing if not the person so aptly reflected by our own golf game?

As Hogan also said, "I learn something new about myself every time I step on the golf course."

Which brings me back to my golf genie. Remember him? When I couldn't make up my mind initially, the genie told me to sleep on it and then make a decision. The next evening, I puffed out my chest and told the genie I wanted straight 300-yard drives forevermore.

He cackled, then slapped me on the back as he handed me the still-smudged golf ball. "Just in case you ever want to talk," he said.

The next day, I played with my usual group of friends. Needless to say, they were shocked, but they seemed to take my newfound prowess well. OK, so one of them took my driver to his radiologist to have it x-rayed. But eventually they stopped complaining.

I was scoring a little lower, but I wasn't necessarily having more fun. It was lonely in the middle of the fairway. I missed looking for balls in the woods with my buddies. I missed the sense of anticipation and nervousness on the tee. The sameness of one perfect tee shot after another was, well, boring.

Far worse, I still plunked approach shots into ponds and bunkers, sprayed them over greens and into the woods. So, in the end, what did I hear, hole after hole?

"Gee, Bill, that's a shame to waste such a great drive." Or "Let's see, 300 yards in one and then four strokes to play the final 100 yards. That's still a bogey."

I tried working on the various parts of my short game, but how could they ever match a perfect drive every time?

They couldn't. I'm not perfect. Frankly, I was miserable.

I waited for a quiet evening, walked to the woods, and rubbed the ball with the smudge on it.

"So how's it going, John Daly?" the reappearing genie said with a chortle.

"Now, that's a fitting comparison," I said, glumly sitting down on a log. "I guess I should have chosen the perfect putter. Or maybe the wedge."

The genie sat next to me.

"There's no perfect choice," he said.

He was right. My genie was just another golf ruse, like a club that won't slice (you'll hook it instead) or a ball that floats to the top of ponds and swims ashore (you'll lose it in the woods).

"Can I have my old golf game back?" I asked the genie.

Smiling, he said, "If that will make you happy, then my work here is done."

I did hold out for a last, minor wish, and here I want you to remember some of the genie's earlier suggestions. I'm not saying what my granted wish was, but if you are playing with me and have a cell phone, you'd better think twice — or hold your belt — before turning it on.

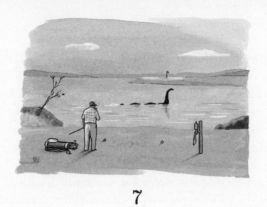

7

Our Biggest Fears

Swinging at daisies is like playing electric guitar with a tennis racket: If it were that easy, we could all be Jerry Garcia. The ball changes everything.

MICHAEL BAMBERGER, *Sports Illustrated*

I'VE BEEN THINKING about how different golf is from a typical holiday or getaway. For example, where do people go when they want to escape or take a break?

Most people head for water. A pristine lake is nice, although something seaside is the most popular choice because people like wiggling their feet in the sand. Some people go camping deep in the woods. And other folks head for bucolic vistas to stare off at verdant rolling hills and lush meadows.

We go to these places because we find the settings relaxing.

Now, think about it. What are the places that golfers universally dread?

Being near water makes them nervous, and hitting over water fills them with panic. No golfer is ever happy in the sand. Heading deep into the woods is almost as distressing. Even gazing out on a vast green vista — like the unspoiled view from the first tee of a golf course — fills most golfers with fear and trepidation.

More proof that while golf may be a metaphor for life itself, it's no vacation.

For the recreational golfer, there are all too many concealed ambushes on the golf course. These are places or situations that lie in wait to embarrass us, test our poise, rattle our nerves, and confuse us with a myriad of choices — none of them seemingly comforting.

We have faced these same situations many times, which doesn't help because that historical knowledge has left us with a burning memory of bad outcomes. Often, the weight of that failure catalog is exacerbated by the apparent simplicity of the task at hand. And yet, over and over we are undone despite our best efforts.

What I'm talking about is the five most feared shots in golf, each one innocent and each one deadly to a golfer's morale and psyche.

What are these round killers?

- Any shot over water, especially one completely over water from tee to green
- A short finesse pitch shot directly over a bunker to a green
- The first tee shot of the day, often executed with a small (or not so small) crowd watching
- Any first, long putt on any green, because it shouts, "Three-putt"
- A recovery shot from the woods — between, around, or below a clump of trees

Maybe you have mastered one or two of these shots. Chances are you haven't mastered most. And even if you have, a bad result still crops up every once in a while. Of course, it would help ease the stress if you had a little strategy to fall back on in these situations.

Sensing that need, and since I have been haunted by these vexing situations as well, I have spent several years seeking advice and counsel from teaching pros, PGA Tour pros, psychologists, and sociologists. Oh, yes, and from bartenders near golf courses, too. But that was in desperation. At any rate, each conversation sought to answer how best to handle these most feared shots.

Playing over Water

Every spring at the seventeenth hole of the Players Championship — the iconic island hole green that is the cynosure of the TPC Sawgrass course — we watch the world's best golfers plunk ball after ball into the water like a bunch of weekend duffers. The tournament has great television ratings, mainly because viewers like to watch pros with perfect swings nonetheless be intimidated by a large expanse of water. It makes them, for a few days at least, just like the rest of us.

On some weekends at the Players Championship, ninety balls find the water.

Don't you just love that?

OK, that's not nice. But the hole is only about 135 yards, and yet the pros fret and fidget on the tee like your brother-in-law squirming to clear a 6-foot creek to win a $5 match. These pros, like average players, know the yardage and know what to do. They have practiced hitting the ball that distance successfully hundreds of times. But just like us, they allow their focus to stray. They see the water. They see shame.

"What's amazing is that if that green were surrounded by sand instead of water, those guys would never miss the green," the coach and teacher Butch Harmon said of the seventeenth hole. "They're such good sand players, it wouldn't faze them a bit. But it isn't sand. So all week at the Players Championship, everyone avoids the subject. Those guys don't even want to talk about it."

So there you have it. It's the water, feared by even the best players.

There is something almost fundamentally dispiriting about a struck golf ball that does not land but instead disappears in a seemingly bottomless lagoon. The ball goes to its figurative death and a little bit of us dies with it. As it descends to the murky depths, our shoulders slump, our knees subtly buckle, and our hopes sag.

Never mind that in most cases, golf's water hazards are but a few feet deep — it's only 4 feet at the TPC seventeenth; to the golfer who once teed up that ball with buoyant aspiration, the ball will sink to oblivion. It's also highly embarrassing. Subconsciously, you can feel your playing partners thinking: "Why'd you hit it there? Didn't you see the water?"

Gary Player, in his quintessential clipped, courtly manner of speech, once talked to me about balls in water hazards. We were seated in a crowded Manhattan bar, but it felt as if he were onstage delivering a Shakespearean monologue:

"Balls splashed in a pond or creek ruin many a round," he said. "And in my experience, they often end up costing more than a lost ball and penalty stroke because they linger in the golfer's mind. They are an arrow that pierces a golfer's collective soul.

"The key is to realize that it is just one shot. And it happens to everyone. And we all play on. Always onward."

Then Gary and I got up, pushed some tables out of the way, did fifty pushups on the floor, and raced each other around two city blocks. (Player is a noted fitness nut.)

Actually, I'm kidding about that part. I ordered another beer while Gary did the pushups and ran around the block.

But Gary is right; rinsing a ball in a pond or lake is like a dagger to the golfing soul. It is one of those "How could you do that to me?" moments that golf doles out with regularity. And because of that, the hitting-over-water problem might seem like a historic or eternal dilemma, but that's not the case. Island greens, or peninsula facsimiles, were hard to find in golf before the early 1980s when Pete Dye designed the TPC course in northern Florida. Pete's wife, Alice, actually gets a major assist for this particular ingenuity. (I guess some might want to blame Alice, but if you met the charming, charismatic Alice Dye — the First Lady of American golf architecture — you would only smile at her cleverness.)

The fact is, the Sawgrass course was a jungle swamp before Pete Dye commenced to push land around with bulldozers. He had framed or staked most of the greens, including the seventeenth green, where he envisioned only a small pond to the right. But the area of the seventeenth green had the best sand on the construction site, and Dye kept borrowing from it to build up other areas of the golf course.

This went on for months until Dye realized that about three-quarters of the land around the seventeenth green was gone. It was Alice, an amateur golf champion and Pete's architecture partner, who while sitting in a cart alongside the proposed tee turned to him and said, "Why not make it an island green?"

And that's what the Dyes did, with only a small 2½-foot-wide walkway connecting the green to the rest of the golf course.

Now, in a typical year, recreational golfers playing the TPC course deposit about 150,000 balls in the lake surrounding the seventeenth green. That's an average of about three balls per golfer (there are 45,000 rounds annually). If that average number of lost balls seems on the high side, you are missing two key points:

Most of the recreational golfers approaching the seventeenth tee have watched many pros fail to reach the green on TV, and that automatically makes the task at hand impossibly intimidating.

Some people, I have been told, will dunk six, eight, or twelve golf balls in the lake, which skews the average.

As daunting a challenge as it has been, the seventeenth hole at TPC Sawgrass has become such a notable golf phenomenon that golf courses have been replicating it by the dozens for the last three decades. But if you don't like this trend, it's not enough just to blame Pete and Alice's design leap.

The truth is that before the advent of better club and ball technology, island greens were not feasible. Before 1980, there might have been only a handful in America. Why?

Because they were considered too hard.

Now you tell us this.

Like many other things in golf, the history of island greens summons a mild dispute. It is not, for example, entirely clear what constitutes an island green. Throughout the last century, it was not unusual for designers to carve small moats around greens, or to redirect a creek into a trough built to envelop a green.

These greens were now technically on islands but maybe not in the sense that most golfers equate with an island green.

"To be what most consider an island green, it should be in a lake or pond or other large body of water," said the golf architect Mike Hurd-zan, a noted golf course historian and author of six books on golf architecture. "And those kinds of greens weren't common at all for many decades."

Hurdzan said true island greens were not a feature borrowed from the centuries of European golf design. He said the ninth hole on the golf course at Florida's Ponte Vedra Inn and Club was generally recognized as the first island green, although there might have been others. The hole at the Ponte Vedra resort, which is not far from TPC Sawgrass, is still in use.

Once again, this being golf, there is always room for another reading of the green, and indeed, there is evidence that the tenth hole on the original course at the famed Baltusrol Golf Club in New Jersey had what was called "the island green." Pictures reveal it as more of a circular green surrounded by a moat. It was a popular par 4, although when the 1904 United States Amateur Championship was played at the course, a delegation of members deemed the island green unfair. An adjacent green was used for play instead.

"The ball used then did not have the aerodynamics that made it fly, and the clubs had a sweet spot about the size of a dime," Hurdzan said. "Golfers were forced to play a lot of shots that bounced and rolled. It was hard to bounce the ball off water."

The Baltusrol island green disappeared in the 1918 rebuilding of the course by A. W. Tillinghast. "During the Great Depression and the World War II years, it's unlikely many island greens were constructed anywhere," Hurdzan said. "No one had the money." Without modern bulldozers, island greens were expensive to construct and posed other logistical issues, like how to get grass mowers and irrigation systems out to the greens.

The consensus is that the next indisputable island green surfaced in 1963 at Golden Horseshoe Golf Club in Williamsburg, Virginia, a course designed by Robert Trent Jones Sr. Jones, incidentally, worked on a redesign at Ponte Vedra in 1947. "The sixteenth hole at the Golden Horseshoe, set in a pond, deserves the credit for introducing the island green concept to designers of the next era," Hurdzan said. In the service of history, I visited the venerable Golden Horseshoe not long ago to play the renowned sixteenth hole, a par 3 of about 155 yards with a tee box looming over the green from an elevated plateau.

Although the green is large, because it is positioned late in the round, it begins to weigh on your mind early in the day. They say the PGA pros at the Players Championship start thinking about the seventeenth hole as soon as they can see it from the tee at number 16. I started thinking about Golden Horseshoe's island green when I put on my golf shoes in the parking lot. I asked for help in the locker room, in the pro shop, and at the snack shack on the course. I even asked advice of the guy impersonating George Washington at nearby Colonial Williamsburg.

But, of course, when that moment comes, you're all alone.

It's just you, the club in your hand, and those quivering knees under your belt.

And all that water.

Glen Byrnes, the director of golf at the Golden Horseshoe, told me a longtime navy officer once said after playing his course's sixteenth hole, "I've seen oceans that looked smaller."

Well, I didn't hit the ball in the water off the tee. But in the spirit of George Washington, I won't tell a half-truth. Afraid of the water and the chance I might hit it fat, I took an extra club and of course hit it flush. It soared over the green until it hit the wooden bridge behind the green that links it to the rest of the course. It bounced far away to solid ground. OK, it still wasn't anywhere near the island green, but I'm claiming a small victory.

As I said, though, I have sought professional advice on how to handle the hitting-over-water situation.

Chuck Cook, rated one of the nation's top ten golf teachers and the coach of several major championship winners, offered this tip:

"Tee the ball up a bit higher, at least the thickness of a full finger above the ground," said Cook, who runs a golf academy at the Barton Creek Resort and Spa in Austin, Texas. "It's a confidence thing because it just looks easier to clip the ball off the tee. Most golfers normally try to hit up on the ball to lift it, which, of course, is the last thing you want to do.

"If it's already teed up, they don't try to lift it. It already looks inviting."

Remember, golf is a game of opposites. If you want the ball to go up, hit down on it.

The late Pat Dolan, a longtime golf pro in Texas who schooled a number of top pros including Lee Trevino, used to tell his students to try to hit the ball into the water with a downward swing as if they were trying to hit a ground ball in baseball. Hitting the ball down, of course, meant a strike that allowed the lift in the club to send the ball into the air — and over the water. So Pat Dolan used to tell his students when faced with water: "Aim for the water."

Try it. You'll be surprised. It works.

Then again, I've heard the opposite advice that makes sense, too. In 2008 in California, I was at a Nike-sponsored clinic Tiger Woods conducted. Tiger told the roughly twenty-five golfers standing around the practice tee that as a young boy he had experienced some trouble with shots over water. He said his father gave him this tip that brought quick success and a lifetime of confidence in the situation:

"My dad said to pick a specific spot on the green to hit to and to really home in on that specific spot," Woods said. "You might not hit that spot, but you'll probably get in the vicinity, at least close enough to be happy with the outcome. But it's essential to have a specific goal in mind. Without a specific goal, most golfers facing water instead think, 'Hit it anywhere but the water.' Or they think, 'Just hit it over the water.' In either case, they are thinking about the water, not the green, not a spot, not the target, not a goal.

"My dad knew that if I focused on the goal, eventually the water would become an afterthought. And it always has been. I might still miss a shot and put it in the water, but only because I missed my target, not because I saw the water."

In other words, imagine if you were shooting free throws in basketball and the first 10 feet from the free-throw line toward the basket was a trough filled with water. Would it make it harder to at least get the ball close to the basket?

Maybe if you had never played basketball or hadn't taken a free throw in ten years, but if you had any basketball experience — sort of like any golf experience — you would focus on the basket and launch the ball toward it. You wouldn't even look at the water.

The mindset, Woods says, should be the same when hitting over water.

There is other advice that seems elementary but few golfers know it or use it. For instance, when you get the yardage for the hole and calculate what is the appropriate club for that distance, take one club longer instead. If you think it's a natural 7-iron, drop down to a 6-iron. This gives you the confidence to swing easy, as opposed to feeling like you must force the swing. The worst thing you can do is think you have to hit it hard to get the ball there. A more patient, relaxed swing is likely if you are sure you have enough club to get the ball over the water.

If this leads you to consistently knock the ball over the green, you can scale back. But more club is a security blanket, and should you suffer from the occasional mishit — not you, I know, but should it happen — extra club might help the ball still clear the water.

David Leadbetter, the noted instructor and former coach to Nick Faldo and Nick Price, tells students at his golf academies to untie their shoes and loosen their belts when hitting over water.

What does that do?

"Untying your shoes promotes excellent balance and good rhythmic weight transfer," Leadbetter said. "It keeps the swing from getting quick in the backswing or the downswing. You have to have a smooth pace. And that's good for any shot on flat ground but certainly suitable to a shot over water."

And loosening the belt?

"Oh, that does nothing," Leadbetter said. "That's just to distract them."

If the students think their pants might fall down, the water is the least of their worries.

Don't you love expert golf instruction?

Finally, as for the old home cure of switching to a cheap ball so you don't worry about losing it: It doesn't work. I have done that dozens of times and almost always put it in the water. It is the ultimate self-fulfilling prophecy. I have found that if I keep the expensive ball on the tee, I'm showing confidence in myself. And there's always the financial incentive, too.

The Finesse Pitch Shot over a Bunker to a Green

If water brings anxiety, then the little 25-yard pitch over a bunker brings a foreboding sense of gloom and a dark capitulation to the inevitable. Your ball may be resting harmlessly in the grass a few yards in front of a greenside bunker, but sizing up this situation, you will make sure to bring along your sand wedge as you approach the ball, even if a sand wedge is not the club you plan to use for the next stroke.

That's because you fear what club you might need next. And it's not a putter. In fact, sometimes you probably forget to bring the putter at all.

What makes this shot hard is again the obvious. Instead of staring at an expanse of water, you can't overlook the sand in your path. You've been told to open your club and swing relaxed. You've been told to shorten your backswing or maybe to lengthen it. You've been told to make a slow, rhythmic downswing or a quick dynamic one. You've been told to use a lob wedge because you're just lobbing it over the bunker. Maybe you've even been told to visualize throwing the ball over the bunker underhand with your right hand. (And maybe you've done this when no one was looking.)

So you've been told a lot of things for what is truly not — at face value — a difficult shot. Still, whatever you've been told, a lot of bad things usually happen, most notably a stubbed chip that strikes the ground behind the ball. It's a shot hit with just enough force to deposit the ball in the sand.

If only there were some simple advice that worked, right?

More than five years ago, Butch Harmon gave me instruction on how to hit this shot. I have used it like magic ever since. I remember his first words to me when I asked for help with this situation: "Oh, that's easy," he said. "You can do it one-handed."

And that's what Butch had me do. About a year later, I found out that his father, the great instructor Claude Harmon, who also won the

1948 Masters, was on the cover of *Golf Digest* demonstrating a version of this lesson forty-five years ago. So was his son in 2000.

It goes like this, in Butch's words:

"Drop about ten practice balls in front of the bunker and take your most lofted club. Now put more weight on your front foot — your left foot if you're right-handed. Not a little weight, more like at least 70 percent. Then take the club with just your right hand and hit down on the ball. The ball just pops up and settles on the green.

"Too many people keep their weight back and try to lift the ball with an upward stroke. That's what causes fat or skulled shots. Once people see how easy it can be with the right technique — weight forward and hit down on the back of the ball — they relax. Just hit down; it'll go up and over."

It works. In any lie.

Yes, I can hear you saying, that might work if I have a decent amount of green to play with. The shot Butch suggests will settle on the green but perhaps with some runout. Granted, that's usually plenty good enough. But what if the situation is more ticklish? What if I have to hit a true flop shot? You know, when there's a bunker between the ball and the green but there is very little green on that side to work with. Admittedly, this is a common amateur golfer problem because we often miss greens on the wrong side, which is to say the side that leaves us with the most trouble to overcome.

Why do we do this? Come on, how do I know? Why do we exist? If Jean-Paul Sartre had played golf, his famous existentialist play *No Exit* would have been about the pointlessness of trying to execute the flop shot over a bunker to a tight, small green.

But since Sartre died in 1980, it's unlikely he ever met Annika Sorenstam (she would have been nine). Annika knows how to get out of this situation successfully. And she has a method you can use as well.

First of all, when I talked to her about this feared shot, she conceded it requires a different technique from the one Harmon talked about.

"I like Butch's advice for most of these kinds of shots, but sometimes you do have to try something that employs a little more touch," she said. "I have three tips or observations."

"Most amateurs play this shot with the ball back in their stance. I suggest playing it forward and keeping your weight and hands back."

"Take the club back slowly but accelerate on the downswing. You must confidently follow through."

"Set up for the shot with the heel of your front foot an inch off the ground. And leave it an inch off the ground as you practice the shot, or maybe as you hit on the golf course. This is to ensure that you do not make a normal transfer of weight from the back foot to the front foot during the swing. That is a good, even essential, move for full shots or chips, but it delofts the club in a flop shot. So practice keeping your front heel off the ground throughout the swing."

A smiling Sorenstam then added, "Make a full finish, and smile when the ball lands soft and safe."

And I would add one more thing. The next time you approach one of these shots, make sure you bring your putter — and only your putter — with you.

First-Tee Jitters

You're on the first tee of a member-guest tournament. You're the guest and your friend's buddies are standing around waiting as you warm up. Already, you feel as if your golf swing is being silently analyzed for proper technique.

You want to do well and the first tee is a symbolic moment. On the practice range a few minutes earlier, you felt smooth and confident, but now the first tee feels a world apart, full of tension and nerves. Worse, you just noticed that the windows of the pro shop and clubhouse dining room face the first tee box.

Is everybody within five miles watching this tee shot? What if you hit a big, embarrassing slice? What if you dribble it?

What if — oh, no — you whiff it?

They call this the first-tee jitters, which sounds a bit wimpy for something so disquieting. In the theater, they give it a beefy name: stage fright. In golf, we ought to call it first-tee terror. It's one of golf's most common maladies, and even the great Tiger Woods has admitted to having it. Trevino once said the only people on the first tee of a PGA Tour event who weren't nervous were the volunteers keeping score. Gary Player says he has meditated on the first tee. Ben Hogan forced himself to slow his every movement.

On the first tee in *Caddyshack,* Rodney Dangerfield tells Ted Knight (aka Judge Smails), "I bet you slice into the woods, $100!"

Responds Knight: "Gambling is illegal at Bushwood, sir, and I never slice."

And we all know what happens.

What's the source of all this angst and edginess? And what can be done about it? It's simply another common staging ground for that continuing golf conundrum. It's almost too easy, which makes it so hard. The ball, after all, is not only not moving, it is propped high on a tee. There is usually not water in the way on the first tee as few designers are that cruel. In fact, designers usually make the driving area on the first tee rather generous. You don't have a score yet — not a single stroke, which also means the whole wonderful day is ahead of you — and yet you feel a subtle but definable pressure. It is typical golf pressure: trying to do the eminently doable.

There is no shortage of advice on how to perform admirably in this setting.

Dana Rader preached a first-tee philosophy I have dubbed "golf avoid-ism." And her first target is the oft-taught pre-shot routine. Rader doesn't mind if you have one, but she believes golfers shouldn't do them standing alongside the golf ball.

"The idea is to keep the mind quiet; you don't want to be having any conversations with yourself standing over the ball," said Rader. "So on the first tee where there's already tension, the last thing you want is to be standing next to the ball for a long time. Get away from the ball, go stand a couple steps behind it, then look at the target and breathe through your nose.

"Think about someplace calm or think about what you're going to do for dinner that night. Take one practice swing. Make everything feel as normal as possible, like you felt on the practice range. Then with a quiet mind, go walk to the ball and hit the shot."

Asked if that produces good results, Rader laughed. "Absolutely," she said. "People thinking about the beach off the first tee always stripe one down the middle."

There were several pros in the don't-linger-over-the-ball camp.

"I tell my students to step on the first tee, take a practice swing about 3 inches from the ball, immediately step closer, and hit it," said Harmon. "There shouldn't be any more thought than that. The other thing I tell them is this: No one watching cares what you do. Golfers are too worried about what other people will think of them. No one cares. The other people are busy worrying about their own first shot."

OK, so it's obvious not letting your mind race is helpful, but is it that easy? Not for everyone, so some teachers had clever tips for defusing the tension.

"I tell people to take in the scenery because the first tee is usually an attractive spot with a view," said Ben Alexander, who operates a golf academy at Poppy Hills Golf Course in Pebble Beach, California. "It's a game, right? Be happy you're out there."

Bryan Jones, director of instruction at the David Glenz Golf Academy in Long Valley, New Jersey, said he encourages students to do a little homework first, making a visit to any golf course to watch other people tee off.

"Take forty-five minutes to watch four or five groups hit off the first tee and you won't be worried about how you look anymore," Jones said. "You might come away feeling pretty good about your ability level."

Eddie Merrins, the charismatic pro at Bel-Air Country Club, has for years advised golfers waiting on the first tee to toss a golf ball a few inches in the air and then catch it. He says it has an almost hypnotic effect when done over and over and promotes a subliminal confidence.

Other teachers felt that first-tee troubles actually start long before the ceremonial first tee box.

"People should eat the right foods in the morning and then get to the golf course early so they're not rushing around," said Kylee Naffziger of the Bridger Creek Golf Course in Bozeman, Montana, who was a finalist for the 2008 PGA Teacher of the Year. "I see people arrive five minutes before their tee time. Would a baseball or basketball player arrive five minutes before a game, hop out of the car, and expect to perform well?"

The overriding consensus was that golfers should warm up on the range slowly, focused on tempo and rhythm only. "It's not the right time to start working on some new tip you received," Alexander said.

I've talked to a few sports psychologists about this situation. Bob Rotella, who wrote the bestseller *Golf Is Not a Game of Perfect* and who remains a fixture on the PGA Tour as a mental guru to dozens of players, preaches clearing your mind and visualizing a straight shot into the verdant landscape. He suggests seeing that shot early, like during the drive to the golf course.

"One thing that works for most people is thinking about tempo," Rotella said. "Slow down. Just try to be smooth or fluid. It's important to try to not overdo anything. Keep your equilibrium."

Rotella had another overriding suggestion.

"Be reasonable and don't make too much of it," he said. "It's just one swing of many that day. Keep it in perspective. Millions of people have shot 75, or better, with a poor first-tee ball."

Dr. Wayne Glad, the Illinois clinical psychologist who has worked extensively with college and pro athletes, including golfers, also believes golfers put too much emphasis on the meaning of the first shot.

"It goes back to people's sense of worth and their ego," Dr. Glad said. "They don't want to lose face or be embarrassed. The first tee shot is very ceremonial in that way.

"But everyone who has ever played golf has hit that shot poorly at one time or another. Golfers understand. Everyone has been there. No one will overly judge you based on what happens on the very first tee shot. So do your best. Stay calm and don't rush it. Hit it and move on. Say to yourself that you will smile afterward regardless of what happens. If you don't make too much of it going in, most likely you will surprise yourself and do pretty well."

And in the end, if nothing else works, be thankful you're not a Tour pro who has to tee off with thousands of people enveloping the tee box.

Tom Joyce, the director of golf at Glen Oaks Club on Long Island, had a long career as a top competitive golfer. He recalled when he made the cut in the 1973 United States Open at Oakmont Country Club. Having made his way through the crowd to start his third round, he arrived at the first tee and saw that fans several rows deep lined both sides of the first fairway. "I said to myself, 'My God, I'm going to kill somebody,'" Joyce told me years ago. "My knees were shaking, and I felt my breathing getting short. And then I just blanked out. I don't remember hitting that ball; I still don't remember it. My muscles took over and knocked it into the fairway."

So there you have it: Hit it before thinking, try hypnosis, or perhaps just blank out. Sounds like golf to me.

Lag Putting, That First Long Putt on a Green

It's really not the first putt that's the problem. It's the putt that's left after the first putt — the one that's too far away to likely go in the hole. The problem with the first long putt is the scary notion that a three-putt is coming. And a three-putt green is the most frustrating outcome in golf. Well, other than four-putting. And that starts with a bad first putt, too.

I have heard all kinds of advice on how to be a better long, or lag, putter. I recall when I was ten years old reading a *Golf Digest* cover story by Jack Nicklaus in which he talked about imagining the hole as having a 3-foot ring around it and your only job was to get the ball inside the 3-foot ring. Sounds simple enough.

If you're Jack Nicklaus.

While short putts are strangely daunting because they are so inherently simple, long putts can be difficult, because let's face it, a lot can go wrong in the 40 or 50 feet you have to get the ball to travel. And yet, if you had to bend down and roll the ball across the green with your hand, you could probably get it fairly close to the hole, especially with practice.

Why is that? The answer is because we would use more instinctual coordination than learned — or overlearned — golf skills. We would be relying on athletic intuition and not the mechanics of the putting stroke. We also allow our eyes to remain focused on the target, and that lets our brain use a steady stream of visual information to get the ball close to the hole. This realization, and the study and understanding of it, is the premise behind a breakthrough putting technique that has already helped many golfers and will probably help many more in the years to come. This putting system, in essence, preaches looking at the hole when you putt instead of looking at the ball. Importantly, it's worth noting that this technique is also based on on-the-green testing with golfers of all handicaps and sound applied athletic science theory.

It does take a leap of faith, but if you keep an open mind, it can unquestionably improve your lag putting. I've tried it successfully for the last several years. But let's start where most golfers start, facing that first long putt on a green.

They size up the putt, and once they get over the ball, they look at the hole several times, turning their eyes from the ball to the hole. Eventually, they fix their gaze on the ball and — eventually — putt the ball in the direction of where they remember the hole to be.

Let's back up and compare this to other sports.

When you play pool, do you look at the cue ball just before a shot or the ball you want the cue ball to hit? If you play basketball, when you are about to take a shot, do you look at the ball in your hands? If you play baseball or softball and have to throw to first base, do you look at the ball in your hand as you're throwing it? Or do you look at the first baseman? If you are playing darts, do you stare at the dart in your hand? Or do you look at the bull's-eye?

OK, so you know where this is going. Now I can hear your questions: "But in baseball or tennis, when I hit the ball I don't look at where I want it to go. I look at the ball." Well, of course you do. In baseball and tennis, the ball is moving, perhaps at seventy or ninety miles an hour. In golf, the ball isn't moving.

The next most common comment is that in darts or in the act of throwing a baseball or softball, the thrown object is in your hand. In golf it is not. Yes, but in golf, you set the putter up against the ball and align yourself right next to it. This is the leap of faith I mentioned earlier. Many people fear that if they take their eyes off the golf ball when putting, it will cause a disastrous mishit.

But what would you think if I told you there was proof that people putt better, even significantly better, when they look at the hole — the target — instead of the ball? What if some of the best golf teachers in the land recommended this method? What if it was by far the easiest way to alleviate the yips and also a cure for chronically poor putting from long distances?

Would you try it?

Chances are you may still think it sounds daffy and you would be embarrassed to try it in front of your friends. Right, as if it's not already embarrassing enough to three-putt four times in one round. And does anyone really need to remind you that putting can account for about 40 percent of the strokes in an average round?

"About 99 percent of my students putt better looking at the hole," Dana Rader, the teacher, told me. "I make all my students try it, and they are amazed. When you look away from the target and stand over the ball for too long, your brain actually loses its memory of how hard to hit the ball. And sometimes where to hit it, too." Because putting prowess may be the most elusive of golf's skills, people have been experimenting with various putting techniques for centuries. But in the last eight years, the effectiveness of looking at the hole while putting has been researched and painstakingly analyzed by Eric Alpenfels, another top-rated instructor and the director of the Pinehurst Golf Academy, and Bob Christina, the dean emeritus of the School of Health and Human Performance at the University of North Carolina, Greensboro.

In 2002, at the behest of *Golf Magazine*, Alpenfels and Christina conducted a field test using forty golfers with a range of handicaps. At the time, Alpenfels and Christina were convinced that people who looked at the hole would putt worse. "These were people who spent twenty or twenty-five years looking at the ball," Christina said. "We gave them forty-five minutes of practice looking at the hole and then started charting and measuring the results. I expected a negative effect."

Instead, golfers of all handicaps putted more effectively. From long distances, golfers looking at the hole hit the ball 24 percent closer. More short putts went in as well, though the improvement was less pronounced. If Alpenfels and Christina weren't convinced at first, they were after they did additional testing over several years. In 2008, Alpenfels and Christina wrote a book, *Instinct Putting,* that summarized their findings and gave a detailed plan of how to convert to what remains an unorthodox approach. Both Alpenfels and Christina emphasized that it didn't take much practice to learn to putt better their way. Christina estimated that golfers would see improvement in forty-five minutes and added, "If they practice more, they will improve more."

Among other findings, Alpenfels and Christina observed that golfers who looked at the hole kept a steadier posture during their stroke. In other words, they were less likely to move their heads, perhaps the most common putting mistake. In addition, people who looked at the hole were less likely to decelerate the putter head before impact — the other major putting mistake. The scientific explanation of why it is more effective to look at the target is that the brain more successfully interacts with the muscles of the shoulders, arms, and hands with a continuous flow of visual information (i.e., the brain knows where the hole is because you are looking at it). But the second you take your eyes off the target, the brain has to interact with the muscles based on its memory of where the hole is. And then there is the aforementioned athletic intuition, which is more likely to come into play when you're looking at the target.

As for the fear of missing the ball with the putter head, it doesn't happen, especially with practice. (I've tried it.) If anything, it's a mental relief not to be tensely staring down, transfixed by ball and putter. But don't take my word for it. Lots of top teachers advocate the method. Even in the ultracompetitive golf instruction market, there has been little or no criticism of Alpenfels and Christina's conclusions. I polled ten of *Golf Digest*'s top twenty golf teachers, and all of them said they believed in the method's merits, especially for very poor putters.

"As a method, it might just be gaining acceptance," said Jim Suttie, a top-ten-rated teacher. "In the future, I think you'll see more people doing it."

So why haven't some top touring professionals looked at the hole instead of the ball? Some pros have tried it, even in competition, most notably Johnny Miller. But that's going back a lot of years. Top pros probably don't try it for the same reason that most recreational golfers haven't tried it. "It is a real leap of faith to look away from the ball,"

Alpenfels said. "It's also relinquishing direct conscious control of the putter head, and that scares people. But when people try it, the result is positive. But it's hard to pull the trigger and try it under the pressure of high-level competition."

I would agree, but most recreational players aren't under that much pressure, and yet we still can't putt. Could we really do that much worse? You don't even have to change your putting stroke. All you have to do is look away from a ball that isn't moving. How hard can it be?

Well, over the years, I've written a few articles in *The New York Times* about this method. In 2010 one of those columns was posted on our "On Par" blog, and some people reacted as if I were proposing we all start putting using a hockey stick while riding a unicycle.

"This cannot work and it would only screw up your putting forever!" a man from Alabama wrote. "It's a gimmick and a hoax."

Wrote Seth from Texas: "Next, you'll tell me to close my eyes."

"You can't compare putting to shooting a basketball — putting is so much more difficult," according to Frank in New Jersey.

And Harold, who said he was a psychologist in Florida, wrote: "Bill, your need to look away from the ball reveals a strong streak of irrational escape-ism or a desire to abandon basic responsibility. Don't do it, Bill; see the ball and hit it."

I think he was kidding. I think. I know from the rest of my mail that most other people were not kidding. They would not dare try looking at the hole. So I agree with Harold that there is something being revealed here — how scared and confused putting renders us. What I saw as most pertinent in these reactions was that so many were ignoring the obvious, which is that the results of the Alpenfels and Christina study reflected years of research conducted, backed up by the experience of dozens of top teaching instructors working in the field. The documented facts are that people do better when looking at the hole. We've all been putting pretty much one way for decades, even centuries, so it is normal for any radical new way of doing something to be opposed and greeted with skepticism. People often don't believe the data or the results of new ideas even though they have not tried the new method. Looking at the hole seems odd and sounds like it won't work — the researchers admitted to the same pre-study belief — but the funny thing is that it does work for most people.

So should everyone who has any difficulty putting — and if people are honest, that is a vast majority of the golfing population — at least try it? Yes, they probably should. Chances are they will be surprised and find it valuable, especially with long putts, or at the very least as a training aid. It's just an idea; give it a try.

Don't make me go get my hockey stick and unicycle.

Playing a Recovery Shot from the Woods

When I began playing golf, I was in the woods so much my golf pro was a raccoon. He was the only one who had seen me swing more than once a hole.

The point is this: If you're going to play golf, unless you are a 5 handicap or better, you are going to spend a fair amount of time in the woods. You might as well get comfortable there. Think of the woods as your friend. Do they not sometimes deflect your very wayward shots back into play? Do they not sometimes knock your opponent's slightly wayward shots far out of play? Do they not offer sanctuary from the heat and bright sun of the fairway?

If you can't bring yourself to think of the woods as your friend, at least stop viewing the woods — and trees in general — as a golfing enemy. Trees are an element we must play with or through, like wind or rain. And every golfer should learn to be at home in the woods, because you're never too good to avoid them forever. And then you need to know how to escape the woods with a good recovery shot.

Don't fear that shot. Learn to deal with it. How? Start by taking a walk in the woods. Preferably, next to a golf hole. That's the advice of Dean Reinmuth, one of the nation's leading teachers and Phil Mickelson's early coach. Keep in mind that Mickelson is one of the best at recovering from the trees that golf has ever seen.

Reinmuth likes to take his students into the woods with a bucket of balls and a few clubs.

"Getting the ball out of the woods and still being in good position is a lot more important than most golfers realize," Reinmuth told me one day near his California home. We were standing, of course, in the woods. "A rescue from this place in the woods is a skill that will save your golf round almost every time you play. When you're in the woods and your next shot hits another tree, or two trees, that's when things start to unravel. The other thing that happens is people hit their shots from the woods too far and get in more trouble. You can eliminate either result with practice.

"I can recall standing in these very woods with a young Phil Mickelson. He was here practicing various recoveries."

So when you watch Mickelson make a miraculous shot like the one he hit out of the pine straw and trees to the thirteenth green on his way to victory at the 2010 Masters, know that he had tried something like that before — probably many times. "Everybody hits bad shots," Reinmuth said. "The difference is that the best players practice for it. But do amateurs?"

You know the answer to that. Average players tend to practice at ranges where the conditions are (usually) uniform. And if they practice on the golf course, they tend to practice from the fairway. Is that realistic?

"You're going to end up behind a tree or a row of trees, and with practice, you might discover that you can still consistently give yourself a chance at par," said Reinmuth, who teaches at the Santaluz golf club in San Diego. "If you can learn how to advance the ball to where you have a nice pitch to the green most of the time, that's worth a lot of shots every round. It begins with accepting and expecting bad shots. It's not always about whether you can hit a 5-iron off a good lie. It might be whether you can hit a 5-iron under a tree branch to a good lie."

It's not about trick shots; it's about experimenting. How does the ball react when you play it back in your stance or forward? What happens when you take a half swing? Or put all your weight on your front foot? We all know we can curve the ball; we do it all the time by accident. But can you do it on purpose?

The answer is yes, but with practice. I'm not talking about one of those insane Mickelson shots where he curves it 50 yards right to left with a 6-iron that goes 200 yards. Most of us cannot learn to do that. I saw Mickelson hitting balls at a range when he was sixteen; trust me, he's not normal. That's a special talent. But you and I can learn to curve the ball 10 yards around a tree for a shot that trundles safely down the fairway another 70 yards. You can learn to do this through trial and error in a practice setting, preferably in actual trees, but it can be done in the perfect conditions of a practice range. Open and close the clubface and alter your alignment. Do what good players do: Practice different things and see what happens. Don't wait to be in trouble to practice getting out of trouble.

There are a few tips some pros have told me over the years. One, from Jim McLean, another top teacher, was to consider choking down on the club. "You can still hit the ball pretty far with your hands down the shaft," McLean said. "But you'll have more control and feel for the shot with your hands closer to the ball."

The other advice that I have found especially helpful came from Joe Hallett, who spent a few years at the PGA Center for Golf Learning and Performance in Florida. Hallett blames a common golf phrase for the trouble people tend to have getting the ball safely out of the woods.

"Every golfer is told to punch it out of the woods," Hallett said. "And they take the term *punch shot* too literally. They slam the ground with their club like a punch. The club either shuts down and the ball stays in the woods, or they pop it up into a tree. What they need to be thinking is that this is a chip shot on steroids. It's just a long chip shot. Feel your arms swing freely. Don't focus so much on the ball; just use a little left-handed backhand motion. Don't tense up and punch it."

My friend Bryan Jones, head of golf instruction at the David Glenz Golf Academy in northern New Jersey, takes students into the woods and has them try to get out of the same spot numerous ways — hitting the ball sideways, backward, around a tree to the right or to the left, under a tree limb, or maybe over it.

"People start walking toward the woods thinking they're in jail," Jones says. "They're defeated before they even get there. It is true that you may have to lower your expectations and take your medicine a little, but you probably have a few very doable options that won't ruin your round."

So don't fear the woods. If you hit your ball there, walk toward it with confidence, as if you're about to visit the living room of an old friend. Just keep the visit with your friend short.

And if you come upon a raccoon who asks about me, tell him I'll give him the $40 I owe him next time I see him. It won't be too long, of that I'm sure.

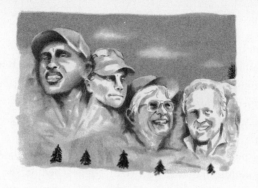

8

Golfing Gods

Lessons Learned Beside Annika, Tiger, and Trevino

There is no such thing as natural touch. Touch is
something you create by hitting millions of golf balls.

LEE TREVINO

I WAS PLAYING golf with Annika Sorenstam a few years ago. We had made some humorous informational golf videos together a few months earlier, and I had covered her competitive career since the mid-1990s. But I had never swung the club in her presence in earnest. She had not seen all the many, varied, well-honed, and impressive parts of my golf game.

After about three shots, Annika turned to me with a puzzled look on her face and asked, "Is that how you always swing, Bill?"

How do you answer such a question? Especially when it's posed by one of the world's great golfers?

I considered: "Well, in fact, Annika, I usually swing much worse."

Or "I'm not sure there's anything in my swing that 'always' happens."

But Sorenstam, who is much too polite to let anyone linger in awkward silence, quickly finished her thought. "I mean, your knees are swaying forward," she said, demonstrating as she talked. "You just don't look very comfortable. Relax, you can make this shot."

I was attempting the long greenside bunker shot, about 70 yards, otherwise known as the hardest shot in golf. And Sorenstam was right; I was neither comfortable nor relaxed. "Get out of the bunker," Sorenstam finally said after I flubbed my attempt to hit the green. "Let me show you."

At this point, Annika had hit exactly one shot, a beautiful drive down the middle of the fairway. With a tight schedule, she had showed up just before our tee time and had not taken any swings beforehand on the range. I'm not sure she had even taken a practice swing before her opening tee shot.

And, the day before, she had announced to the world that she was pregnant with her first child.

But now she stepped into the bunker. She dropped a ball in the sand. It wasn't even a good lie. Again, with no practice swing, she swung her sand wedge. She barely contacted the sand, picked the ball clean, and deposited it 8 feet from the hole 70 yards away. She shook her head as if she were thinking: "I can do better than that."

She dropped two more balls, and as she was talking about how to play the shot, she swung twice more. Now there were three balls about 8 feet away.

Sorenstam stopped and she apologized for the results. "I'm still a little stiff," she said. "I haven't played in a while."

My response was different: "That was ridiculous. How did you do that?"

Sorenstam smiled.

"People think too much about the sand in the bunker," she said. "If you had a 70-yard shot from the fairway, you could do it, right? So before you get in the bunker, take a practice swing on the grass, then get into the bunker and use that same swing. Don't even think about the sand."

I said, "It's not that easy for us regular people."

She replied, "Train your brain."

Then came one of the chief revelations of the day. I asked, "How many times have you practiced this shot?"

Annika laughed. "Oh, I don't know," she said, walking away. "Thousands of times."

That reminded me of a story Sorenstam tells at clinics. In the last few years as I have gotten to know her better I have been fortunate to go to a bunch of them. As she tells the story, it was a rainy day when she was a young teenager in her native Sweden. She called her father, Tom, and asked him to pick her up early at the golf course. When she got in the car, her father saw that other young golfers were still on the range, practicing in the rain.

"When we were inside the car," Annika says, "my father turned and said, 'You know, Annika, there are no shortcuts to success.'"

I relate this story not to explain how our golfing gods are able to do what they do. The message is not that they have just practiced more than the rest of us. Anyone who has been around professional athletes doing anything athletic knows they are unusually gifted. Certainly, there are exceptions, but most can usually beat the average person at most athletic activities — table tennis, billiards, darts, free-throw shooting, or jumping on one leg with their eyes closed.

Sorenstam, for example, was also once a ranked junior tennis player before she concentrated on golf, and she is still an expert skier. Her success, like that of other pro golfers I have played with — Tiger Woods, Lee Trevino, and Phil Mickelson — is in part a result of her advanced athleticism. But it is more than hard hours of practice and innate talent. There is another piece to the combination of skills that sets them apart. In Sorenstam's case, I have seen the evidence of it more than once.

In 2003, I knelt behind the first tee as Sorenstam prepared to tee off at the PGA Tour's Colonial Open. She was about to become the first woman to play in a PGA event in fifty-eight years. Babe Didrikson had done it last, in 1945, but there had not been hundreds of reporters chronicling the scene. Didrikson's opening tee shot was not carried on live national television.

Two weeks earlier, Vijay Singh had summed up the response of many of the PGA players at the time: "She doesn't belong out here." Singh said he would withdraw from the tournament if paired with Sorenstam. He added: "I hope she misses the cut."

It was more than a tense, pressure-filled scene on that first tee that day. It was riveting, heart-thumping drama. Sorenstam emerged from the locker room looking more pallid than usual. She had spent the last thirty minutes sitting alone in the women's locker room, while every other competitor had been mingling in the men's locker room. Sorenstam waited out her tee time in seclusion. Fans cheered her arrival on the first tee. Meanwhile, I noticed she kept taking exaggerated deep breaths. Sorenstam's opening tee shot split the middle of the fairway, and as she began walking toward it, her knees slumped and she patted her heart as if pretending to faint.

Later that week, I asked Sorenstam how she managed to perform in that setting, when she would have been forgiven for a case of first-tee jitters gone awry.

"I told myself that there was nowhere else on Earth I wanted to be at that moment," she answered.

Keep in mind that this is a person who as a junior golf player was so shy she would purposely three-putt the final green in tournaments, so she would finish second, and avoid having to make a speech when accepting the winning prize.

"But you looked awfully nervous; what about the pressure?" I asked.

"I was a wreck, are you kidding?" she said. "My hands were trembling as I stuck the tee in the ground. But again, I wanted to be there. I said: 'Trust yourself. You know how to hit this shot.' So I did."

"Just like that," I said.

"No, it was really hard," Annika said. "But I was determined to do it."

A few years later, I got to see a different side of how a champion walks the golf course in competition. And I discovered that top golfers are plagued by the same vexing doubts and worries that consume average golfers. To see what it's like inside the ropes, I volunteered to be a standard-bearer at an LPGA tournament in Maryland. That responsibility is thankfully not as august as it sounds. The standard-bearer is the person who walks behind the competitors carrying an oversize sign with the players' scores. I pulled some strings and got assigned to Sorenstam's group.

"Don't drop that on my foot," she said on the first tee. It would have all been very funny had I not had to sneeze moments later as Sorenstam stood over the ball, getting ready to hit her first shot. I barely suppressed it, sneezing just after she struck the ball. "Bless you," she said, and marched after her ball. My education was just beginning.

I learned a lot being a few feet from pro golfers playing for a lot more money than most of us ever do. First, their outings are nothing like the foursomes we play with. For example, even though they take a lot of time to line up putts and each has pre-shot routines, they play a lot faster than us because they hit far fewer shots. It was also notable how polite, serene, and quiet the game was in the close company of top players. From 50 yards away and behind the ropes, the spectators had little inkling that the players were talking softly in the middle of the fairway, where they almost always were. What the fans missed were the most carefree conversations about nothing: the weather, sunglasses, the drive to the course, a new pair of shoes. They laughed but rarely grimaced at a poor shot.

I noticed that some social graces transfer regardless of the setting. When one of Sorenstam's playing partners, the New Jersey–bred pro Diana D'Alessio, visited the restroom next to one tee, Sorenstam waited for her. It was as if they were having dinner at a restaurant and Sorenstam didn't want D'Alessio to trudge 250 yards by herself to catch up with the group. I could not imagine that happening in my regular foursome. Or the PGA Tour for that matter. The professional men are far more self-absorbed. And a bit more cutthroat. As Arnold Palmer said, "I never rooted against an opponent but I never rooted for him either."

So the LPGA players were more communal if still very serious — walking fast and sweating — and the import of the proceedings was forever evident. After each golfer missed a short putt on one of the last holes, Sorenstam and her two playing partners all looked perturbed. At the next tee, they were forced to wait for the group ahead of them to clear the fairway. On the cramped tee box, a full five minutes passed with no one — not the caddies, not the players, not the volunteers — saying a word. Spectators peered back up the fairway at the group, anticipating the shots. On the tee, all you could hear were crickets, the babble of a nearby brook, and a far-off train horn.

Sorenstam did not play particularly well that day, and when I went to find her afterward, she was on the practice green, rolling in 6-foot putts. She had three balls at her feet, and when she filled the hole with them, her caddie would pull them out and roll them back to her. I knew not to interrupt her practice. I decided to wait. I gave up after fifty minutes. Tom Sorenstam's daughter was still not cutting any corners.

A few months later, we were shooting another video on how to chip effectively from just off the green, about 30 yards from the hole with nothing but the green's collar and a little swale in our way. This is when I got another look at what it's like to be with *them,* the golf immortals who play and work inside the ropes.

"Amateur golfers make this shot too hard," Annika said. "They would do much better if they would free their minds on the golf course and just try to execute each shot simply. Don't complicate something you could do easily if you were playing alone."

So with our cameras rolling for the video, I used a sand wedge to loft the ball near the hole. Sorenstam stepped up next and urged me to hit a bump-and-run shot from the same spot with a 7-iron instead. She then demonstrated. But on the first try, her ball settled about 6 feet from the hole and a foot farther away than my attempt.

Turning to me, she said, "Nice job." But quickly she added, with a little feistiness, "Let's do it again."

We did five more takes for the video, each of us trying to hit it close. Sorenstam, eyes narrowing, nearly sank every ball she struck. She hit the flagstick a couple of times, and no shot stopped more than 2 feet from the hole.

Suffice it to say, my ball was never inside hers again.

"So you're telling me that was simple?" I said.

"It was simple," Sorenstam replied. "I used a putter stroke with that 7-iron and aimed a little more left after I saw the break in the green. Very simple."

But what about that look of determination I saw in her face?

"Determination helps, yes," she said, laughing. "But it is not tense determination. Focus is good, but take a deep breath and believe in yourself. Relax; it's a game."

Easy for her to say, I know.

Being around Annika Sorenstam, and other golf stars, has convinced me that top golfers play exactly like their developed, or innate, personality. In the end, the essence of who they are cannot be obscured in their golf game. Their golf game is who they are. You probably could say the same thing for most of us. When I played that first round of golf with Sorenstam, we squeezed in another video shoot afterward. It took place on the practice range. It was about hitting the driver, and Annika started hitting one perfect drive after another.

Her swing was smooth and unforced. The power of it kind of snuck up on you. There was a little hip and big shoulder turn, then *bam!* And the ball rocketed down the fairway. Her tempo was even and steady, and her movements serious but not showy. And finally, there was an unquestionable athleticism and a lot of practiced strength that came from the core.

I stood there for a few minutes as she fired shot after shot straight into the sky. Finally, I couldn't resist. I had a question.

"Is that how you always swing, Annika?" I said.

Tiger Woods glared as I stood over my ball on the tee box, his dark eyes giving me that unnerving death stare that has melted the resolve of professional golfers worldwide. I returned his gaze and tried to appear unmoved, an ineffective ploy because the rest of me was shaking.

I was competing as a guest in an event called Tee It Up With Tiger, in which two dozen ordinary golfers got a chance to play a hole with Woods at the Trump National Golf Club outside Los Angeles. It was November 2008, and I had been waiting months. Now Woods watched from about 8 feet away.

Planning for this moment, I had hoped to avoid nervousness by relying on my pre-shot routine. But who among us has a pre-shot routine for hitting in front of Tiger Woods?

As I looked at the ball, all that came to mind were the conversations I had had the night before with the other average golfers.

"We all fear the same thing," said Jeremiah Christy, a government contractor from Maryland. "We don't want to dribble it off the tee. Everyone is praying, 'Please, God, let me get the ball airborne.'"

So this was the day when Joe the Golfer played with Tiger Woods. The lucky twenty-four were winners of a sweepstakes sponsored by

Nike Golf and *Golf Digest* magazine. Two thousand platinum-colored Nike One balls had been randomly distributed in unmarked containers to retail outlets and clubs nationwide that year. Those who bought one of those balls qualified to enter the sweepstakes, as did a select number of golfers who registered online.

"When I found that platinum ball, it was like finding the gold ticket in a Willy Wonka bar," Christy said.

This was, of course, before the infamous Thanksgiving night auto accident in 2009 that eventually unraveled Tiger's world. When I stood before him, golf, in its entirety, was still wholly his kingdom.

On that 2008 day, the winners who claimed those platinum-colored golf balls represented twenty states. They were whisked to the Trump course along the Pacific Ocean. Originally, Woods was going to hit shots on one hole with every foursome, but knee surgery after his win at the U.S. Open at Torrey Pines had limited his mobility and prevented him from taking full swings. Instead, Tiger agreed to accompany every group on Trump National's tenth hole, where he gave advice before and after shots, read greens like a caddie, and hit greenside chip shots. He also relished making fun of some swings and their results. He announced this ahead of time: Dump one in the ocean or skull your ball across the ground and Tiger was going into full trash-talking mode.

Hence, the added apprehension.

My group had begun play on the second hole, which gave us almost two hours to anticipate what everyone was calling "the Tiger Hole." Acknowledging the manifest anxiety, I started spraying shots all over the course right away. Alongside me, Ken Piety, an engineer from Knoxville, Tennessee, was coolly hitting some towering irons. He looked ready. Ed Fillbach, a beginning golfer and semiretired painting contractor from Belgrade, Montana, struggled a bit on the tough course but kept smiling.

The best golfer in the group, Brett Wright, was hitting the ball 285 yards off the tee with a beautiful draw. He also stopped at the eighth tee to order a double Captain Morgan and Coke from the cart girl.

"Something to calm the jitters," said Wright, who works for the Federal Reserve in Memphis.

As if the situation needed more pressure, the Golf Channel was there shooting video for a three-episode show to be broadcast the next week. When we approached the tenth tee, we saw it was surrounded by about thirty camera operators, technicians, and photographers.

Tiger greeted everyone with a beaming smile and a vigorous handshake. He wore a light blue shirt, khaki shorts, and white sneakers. He waved his hand toward the ocean and playfully apologized for the poor weather and the bad view. (It was about 90 degrees, and the vista from the elevated tee was stunning.)

"God, I miss the SoCal weather," he said.

This was not the Tiger Woods I had been around in tournaments throughout the past decade. There was no stoicism. He giggled and asked questions. He wanted to know where my playing partners lived and what they did. Fillbach is from Montana, a place Tiger had never been. That sparked an exchange about mountain golf and playing in locales where the winters are long and the golf season short.

"I don't think I could have grown up like that," Woods said. "I know my dad would have moved us away."

"Maybe," Fillbach said. "But he would have missed out on a whole lot of good fishing."

It was like being at a barbecue.

Then it came time to hit a shot, and Tiger's smile evaporated. The hole is a 280-yard par 4 with a green on a plateau above a gaping chasm that juts toward the ocean. For this event, the tee had been moved up to about 190 yards, and you had to hit it nearly that far to carry the gorge and some bunkers.

"It's playing about 205 yards," Tiger said solemnly. He conceded that he had seen many shots lashed into the wild brush of the chasm.

"But there have been some good shots," he said. "All you have to do is get the ball up there against the wind about 200 yards and let it land soft."

Then, unsmiling, he stepped back.

Thanks. Nothing to it.

Fillbach went first and stroked the best shot he had hit all day, but it landed short in the brushy ravine. He really came through with a good shot, and I was proud of him. I think he was proud, too. It's golf; things don't work out sometimes even when you do your best.

Wright, perhaps feeling his Captain Morgans, drilled a shot to the very back left of the green, maybe 60 past the hole. He seemed relieved. Asked later what he had been thinking, Wright said, "I noticed for the first time that I was taller than Tiger."

Piety smacked his shot directly into the high grass 40 yards from the tee. It never got more than a few feet off the ground. It was a skulled laser.

"At least it was straight," Tiger said, laughing.

Piety had played the previous eight holes in about one over par. "Really, I was playing great," he pleaded to Tiger, who nodded, grinned, and added, "Sure. But you're not getting a mulligan."

We've all been there. And trying to explain that you're really not as bad as that one shot makes you look doesn't really do any good. It's golf; even when you're a good player, things sometimes don't work out. Besides, it was easy to be off your game with Tiger standing there giving you the death stare. It had thrown off many a top golfer; now it was doing the same to us Average Joes.

So finally it was my turn. Woods stood behind me, his arms sternly folded across his chest.

Surprisingly, I did stay in my customary pre-shot routine. I did not pause over the ball for an extra second or two or think about what this swing meant to my day. My only thought was not to rush my backswing, to let the swing have a rhythmic tempo — a full backswing and a full downswing.

Oh, let's face it, the truth is I was shaking with nervousness and finally I just swung.

But I will say that I had prepared in one clever way. Knowing the length of the Tiger Hole beforehand, I had decided I was going to hit my 5-wood, one of my favorite clubs. So on the ninth hole, the last before we met up with Tiger, I teed off using my 5-wood even though it was a long par 4 that normally would have called for a driver. And since that tee shot still left me about 200 yards to the hole, I hit the 5-wood again, landing it on the ninth green.

So by the tenth tee, my 5-wood and I were on pretty comfortable terms. Still, I had never hit a shot with the top-ranked golfer in the world, a few Golf Channel cameras, and maybe another thirty strangers watching.

So when I did eventually swing, I waited to look up, not being in a rush to receive bad news.

"That's a good shot," Woods said. And we watched together as the ball worked a little right to left, struck the right side of the green, and stopped 35 feet from the hole. I was so happy that I didn't chunk it I forgot that we had a cart and started walking toward the green.

Tiger, who had his own cart, pulled up alongside me.

"What are you doing? Are you walking so you can get more camera time?" he said. "Get in the cart."

So we rode to the green together. I asked him what he would have hit from that tee.

"Six-iron," he said. "Got to take the wind into account. And the firmness of that green."

He looked at me. "Why?" he said. "What did you hit?"

"Five-wood," I answered. "Got to take a mishit into account. And the weakness of my overall body structure."

So I got a laugh out of the golfer with the death stare.

Up at the green, Tiger pulled the flag and squatted to line up my right-to-left downhill putt. We stood together for a while, then he walked away and pointed to a small mark about 20 feet from the hole, instructing me to roll my ball over that spot.

"Yeah, but how hard do I hit it?" I asked.

"Do you want me to do everything for you?" Tiger replied.

Part of me was just happy to have found the green at all. But as I stood over the ball, I remember thinking that a three-putt would really ruin a good tee shot. Not to mention a good story. But fortunately I did not dwell over the ball, and after I putted it, I thought it would probably be pretty close. Until it fell in the hole.

With the tenth hole set up like a long par 3, that meant I had made birdie, although a course official later told me, "The scorecard says the tenth is a par 4; that's an eagle."

Tiger came over and shook my hand, holding it for a few seconds.

"Nice putt," he said.

I blurted out the only answer that came to mind: "I think you made the right read on that putt."

And Tiger Woods shot me a look that seemed to say, "I've done this before, you know."

Then he smiled, wished us luck, and headed back to the tee for the next group. We played for the next couple of hours in the sun and by the sea. I don't recall if I got another ball airborne all day. And I didn't care.

After the round, Tiger conducted a clinic for us on the practice range with Anthony Kim, who had arrived via helicopter. Even though I have covered professional golf for years, as I stood a few feet from Woods and Kim — this time without a crowd of thousands surrounding them and without the long stretches of empty fairway that make anyone seem larger than life — I was once again struck by how small some of these guys are.

Nick Faldo, Ernie Els, and even Mickelson, those are fairly big guys. Kim can't weigh more than 155 pounds. He is 5-10 at best. That's about my size. But Kim hits his driver on average 70 yards farther than I do. He hit 7-irons with one hand to demonstrate the importance of tempo and still they traveled 175 yards. He threw a ball into the air, let it strike the ground, then hit it with his 3-wood on the bounce about 250 yards. And it was struck arrow straight.

Oh, yes, and he added that he was a little off his game because he hadn't touched his clubs in three weeks.

Woods, meanwhile, is just 6 feet, 185 pounds. But he wasn't putting on any shows of power. He was resting his knee. So instead he put a regular range-ball pail about 20 yards away. He said he would make ten attempts to chip a ball into the pail and wanted those of us watching to guess how many he would make. The ball had to go in and remain in the pail, not just glance off it.

The general consensus was three balls in the pail. And you could tell most of us were just trying to be nice with those predictions. Tiger wasn't impressed. He told those of us who expected the total to be less than five to put a dollar on the practice range near his feet. Most of us did, myself included. One wise guy said he would give Tiger $20 if he made six or more.

And we all whooped and laughed.

Tiger made the first two, missed two, made two more, missed one, then made another one. That gave him five in the pail with two shots to go. He missed the next one, then lofted the last shot right into the middle of the pail. As he scooped up the dollars, he turned and scanned the crowd: "Where's my $20?"

He collected that money, too, and he quickly put it in the pocket of his shorts.

It was a stark contrast to the Woods the rest of the world would so intensely scrutinize almost exactly a year later. I've come to think of that day as one of the last unguarded and public displays of Woods at play. The window to his life and his thoughts may never be that open again.

And yes, there were several golf lessons learned. That day several people had been curious how Woods and Kim went about warming up for a golf round. This is probably because for most of us squeezing a ketchup bottle over a hot dog qualifies as an adequate warm-up for eighteen holes.

Not surprisingly, Woods is methodical. Remember I said a golfer's game reflects his or her personality? No different here.

Tiger's warm-up commences with first hitting his sand wedge, then his 8-iron and his 4-iron. He typically moves to a fairway wood, then his driver. Then he works his way back down the ladder in his bag, filling in some gaps: 5-iron, 7-iron, 9-iron, and pitching wedge. The last thing he does before he leaves the practice range is hit the club he knows he is going to use on the first tee, whether it's his driver or a 2-iron.

It all sounded so meticulous, like a NASA space shuttle pre-launch protocol, but the major revelation might have been somewhat the opposite. It was revealing how much pro golfers adapt their games based on how their warm-up sessions are going.

"In any warm-up on the range, you should see what shots you have that day," Woods said. "If you're hitting fades, don't fight it; go out and play fades."

Kim added: "You have to play with what you got that day. You don't do it right away, but if I see a trend, I'll adjust my stance, my ball position, my aim — whatever — to the ball flight I'm seeing off the club. I don't try to overcome it; I don't have that much time."

The warm-up, Woods said, is no time to work on swing technique. It is a warm-up, not a lesson, and not a practice session.

"I might be hitting 10-yard hooks or 10-yard fades, but I'm going to go with it for as long as that's the pattern," he said.

Woods, of course, does not hang around too many public course ranges, where the question would be: How do you play with a 50-yard slice? Which is something I brought up to Tiger.

"Find something on the range that is working — a 3-wood or a 5-wood or a hybrid — and play that for a while," he said. "Then you can come back to the driver, or whatever club it is you might need. But if you start with something that wasn't working on the range — a club you clearly have little confidence in at that moment — your day is only going to get worse.

"Don't try to make those fixes on the range. Try to go with what you do have working. Then, an hour into your round when you're relaxed, try hitting your driver again."

It's a point well taken. The warm-up session is like a mini test drive of the car you're renting for the day. It's no time for an engine overhaul.

As a father of children who play golf, I also wondered how Woods, who I think we can agree was a pretty fair junior player, would instruct young beginning golfers on the basics of the game. Like, for example, how hard to swing.

"Obviously, you can't tell an eight-year-old to swing at 85 percent of normal," Woods said. "An eight-year-old doesn't know how to gauge something like that in the middle of a swing. So when I was young, my father told me that I could swing as hard as I wanted, just so long as I was in complete balance when I had finished my swing.

"At the end of a shot, I couldn't be swaying side to side, falling back, or lurching forward. I had to be in balance. I still think it's a great tip: Swing as hard as you like so long as you can be in balance. It puts you in charge of managing the speed and pace of your swing."

Of course, that works not only for junior players. It would work, most likely, for everyone.

Woods also went out of his way to assure his audience that they should not be ashamed to have a shot-saving club like a 7-wood in their golf bags. Same thing for two or three hybrid clubs.

"I now have a senior club in my bag," Woods said. "It's a 5-wood. I'm OK with my senior club."

He looked right at me and smiled.

"I saw a couple of good shots out there today with senior clubs," he said.

Thanks a lot, I thought. Don't you know I made eagle?

Tiger continued: "When I was a teenager, I hit a 1-iron," he said. "Then I moved down to a 2-iron. So now that I'm in my thirties, I've got the 5-wood. When I'm in my forties, it will probably be a 7-wood. A decade later, it'll be a 9-wood. And in my sixties, I'll probably be playing an 11-wood. I have no shame; this game is too hard."

After the clinic, Woods sat down for a forty-five-minute question-and-answer session with Jaime Diaz of *Golf Digest*, who has known Tiger since he was sixteen. Golfers in the audience asked questions as well, some about his personal life. Tiger was not highly revealing.

Over the many years I've been around Tiger I've come to the conclusion that his reticence to talk about his life off the golf course — both before the scandal and after it — is a sincere response. An honest Tiger Woods reaction is a defensive one.

Jaime Diaz told me that in his first meeting with Woods, a sixteen-year-old Tiger said he would never tell reporters what he was thinking.

So a guarded Woods is a genuine Woods. To me, it doesn't make him unlikeable; it's just who he is. Surprisingly, as much as I had watched him for years, and as close as I got to him in afternoons spent at his golf clinics, I really came to understand Tiger in the many hours I spent with him during his disastrous 2010 season, when his every movement got very complicated and his game deserted him.

When Tiger made his return to competitive golf at the 2010 Masters, it was my assignment to follow him wherever he went from the time he stepped onto the Augusta National Golf Club grounds — often just after dawn — until he left the club, usually about ten hours later. I did this for eight consecutive days. I was on the Tiger beat. Heck, I was the Tiger beat. While assorted reporters followed Tiger from time to time, I'm not aware of anyone else who tracked his every movement nonstop. I was either determined or demented.

What is to be learned in this kind of setting? On the day of his first Masters practice round, spectators greeted him with an eerie silence. The whir and rumble of two helicopters filming Woods overhead was nearly all that could be heard, and when the helicopters finally moved on, people stared at him but did not react. As he walked to most tee boxes, the galleries parting to let him pass did so entirely without comment. By his first competitive round later in the week, the crowd cheered him when he made a good shot but not with the gusto and unabashed zeal that they had before his marital scandal. There were occasional snide remarks shouted about his serial adultery, which Woods outwardly ignored even if you could see in his eyes that he had heard them. His jaw would also clench and you could see the tension in his face. From my vantage point a few feet away, it seemed to affect him. Tiger's trademark precision and uncanny calm on the greens, for example, were gone. Short putts he would have made in his proverbial sleep did not drop. Easy chips were mishit just enough to lead to another bogey. Tiger was waging war with par and his critics, and no one wins that battle. By the last round, when it was clear he wasn't going to win the tournament, the fans still cheered him. They were glad he was present and maybe they pitied him a bit, which was an amazing realization when you consider that just six months earlier he had been the world's best-known and perhaps most respected athlete. To me, on the last day I felt as if the fans who cheered did so because they missed the old Tiger more than they appreciated the reappearance of this new Tiger.

It was all a bit lonely, but it was also clear Woods was seeing and taking in everything around him. All the clamor and turmoil had not changed his renowned focus, attention to detail, and powers of observation — something I discovered firsthand. Toward the end of the third round on Saturday, as he was completing the thirteenth hole — I had now been following him for forty-nine consecutive holes plus three practice rounds — I had to visit the men's room. I ducked away from Tiger's detail, which included some reporters and four security officers. In the process I missed him play the fourteenth hole.

So to catch up, I used some of the course knowledge gained from my sixteen trips to Augusta National. With a shortcut through the pine straw and loblolly pines, I dodged the voluminous crowds and hurried ahead to the fifteenth tee, getting in good position alongside the tee box, where I knelt and waited. As Tiger and his caddie, Steve Williams, finally made their way to the fifteenth tee, Tiger walked past me. He turned his head, looked me in the eye, and said: "Where did you go?"

More than a little surprised, I sputtered: "To the bathroom."

He grinned. "OK, just wondering," he said.

Woods was in the middle of thousands of fans, in the middle of a week of media mayhem — and still in contention for the tournament — and he had an airplane circling the golf course dragging a sign that read, SEX ADDICT? YEAH. RIGHT. ME TOO!

This was his new world. And yet he saw it all. And he still wanted to make a joke if he could.

A couple of months later, I was no longer tethered to his side as the United States Open was contested at the Pebble Beach Golf Links, but I still saw the isolation that had grown around the man and his golf game. On the Wednesday morning before the first round of the tournament, one of the strangest sights at the practice putting green was Tiger Woods, alone.

There was no caddie, no coach, no agent or press attaché. It had been a long time since Woods was found alone at any tournament. Once he would have been surrounded by a doting entourage that included security. On that Wednesday, it was just Woods working on his game for the United States Open with a putter and four balls. Woods had not won a tournament in nine months, and much of his inner circle had been disrupted by the scandal. A month earlier he had split with longtime coach Hank Haney, and caddie Steve Williams was now something less than the competitive soulmate he once was. (Their partnership would end in about a year.)

So on this day at Pebble Beach, in solitude, Woods had to attend to little things that in the past were done for him by a coach or caddie, whether it was retrieving his balls from the hole or putting his tees in the ground for one of his favorite putting drills. (The tees are positioned like goalposts so that Woods's putter head barely passes through them during his stroke.)

Woods's fellow competitors gave him a wide berth, leaving him in a remote corner of the large putting surface. There were seven or eight other golfers practicing in clusters, and then there was Woods, as if separated by an invisible force field.

Rory McIlroy, the youngster from Northern Ireland, looking small and wide-eyed next to Woods, dared to penetrate his space. He wandered over and made small talk, slapping Woods on the back as both laughed. But McIlroy retreated after a few minutes, and Woods again moved from putt to putt, silently and unaccompanied.

Stranger still, as he putted, Woods was being watched by about 200 fans, who aimed cameras at him and strained three and four deep against a nearby railing. The dynamic between Woods and fans remained as complicated and odd as it had been at the Masters. In his presence, the fans said nothing — no words of encouragement, no catcalls. There was not even the usual murmuring heard in such settings when a long putt drops in the hole or just misses it. It was so quiet it felt as if people were holding their breath, not sure what to do or what to say, but certain they were not supposed to contribute to the scene.

The fans at times were no more than 6 feet away but remained still and mute, staring at Woods as they might at an exhibit in an art gallery. Woods did not return their gazes or break the hush.

He was working, and every putt was not rolling into the hole. He would shake his head, pluck the balls out of the hole, drop them again, and continue.

Occasionally, he muttered to himself, little statements that no one but him heard.

Woods did not win that event either. But watching him that day — and comparing him to the jovial Tiger of just a year earlier — I thought it was crushingly evident how much he had lost.

Lee Trevino was hitting balls into a net in the garage of his Dallas home. Sixty-four years old at the time, Trevino still did this for hours.

He would do it more often but his back doesn't allow it. Trevino was talking about the golf clubface.

"You know what is the most misunderstood thing in golf?" he asked without looking at me. "Everyone wants to talk about swing plane, hip turn, weight shift, and the X-factor."

Trevino was swinging as he talked. He would start a sentence:

"And meanwhile, the single most important thing . . ."

At this point, he would take the club back in that inimitable outside-in loop of his and pause.

"Is the clubface . . ."

He would then complete his swing, contacting the ball in the center of the clubface. Trevino stopped to lean on his club (a favorite pose).

"But does anyone talk about the clubface?" he asked. "Don't answer that. Because I'll tell you. The answer is 'No.' The clubface is the man. You know when guys yell after a shot, 'You da man!'? That's who they are talking to — they're talking to the clubface."

Trevino was going to give a clinic the next day, and he was showing me the shots he was going to hit. He explained, then demonstrated how he was going to curve the ball left to right, then right to left, then low to high, then high and soft. He said he would hit some shots that did seemingly impossible things, like curve 40 yards and hit a single tree. He never stopped talking as he did this.

Trevino's history is well known: a Dickensian childhood in Dallas at a home with no electricity or running water that happened to be near the seventh hole of a private golf course. He picked cotton as a child, later became a caddie, worked at a driving range, taught himself to play golf, and left school in the eighth grade.

"But I did go to college," Trevino said. "I delivered a Christmas tree to SMU every year."

The golf range, likened to the one in the movie *Tin Cup*, was converted to a Christmas tree stand every winter.

He enlisted in the Marines at seventeen, which he said toughened him for life.

"Drill instructor punched me in the face fifteen minutes after I got there," he said. "I just got back up and stood at attention."

He kept playing golf as a Marine, and since he was a good, bet-winning partner of officers on the golf course, he got to play a lot. When he returned to civilian life, he became a club pro. With a wealth of determination, he made it to the PGA Tour in 1967 and was named Rookie of the Year. But his swing was so unorthodox people called that season a fluke. In his second year, he won the U.S. Open, the first of six major championships.

As Trevino said: "My first year on tour I told all these jokes as I walked around the golf course and people ignored me. No one laughed at all.

"The next year, after I won the U.S. Open, I told the same jokes and everyone laughed themselves silly."

In the years I followed Trevino's career — admittedly most of the in-person sightings were during his wildly successful senior tour career — he always seemed like the perfect guy for amateur golfers to emulate. But in general, that wasn't the case. Everyone loved the Merry Mex, but for the most part, regular golfers wanted to swing like Jack Nicklaus or Tom Watson.

"I am the regular golfer," Trevino once said, pleadingly. "I'm the digger, the grinder. I had average golf skills and a messed-up swing to start. I just worked harder."

What Trevino honed over many hours, among other things, was the ability to control the clubface. And indeed, at several tournaments and at clinics I saw Trevino conduct over the years, he could do almost unfathomable things with a golf club and a golf ball. The day after that afternoon in his garage, at the clinic he was prepping for, he did point at a pine tree about 150 yards away.

"I'm going to aim 40 yards left of that pine tree, then hit a big sweeping fade that smacks the tree about halfway up the trunk," he said.

When he missed the tree by about 2 feet on the first try, he apologized. His next try hit the trunk of the tree with a loud *thwack*.

Trevino went on like this for thirty minutes, describing the shape of the shot he was going to hit for the folks in attendance, then performing it faultlessly, the balls curving in different directions against the blue sky as if Trevino were drawing their trajectories with a pen.

I recalled an old Trevino quote: "I used to be able to hit a 2-iron through a doorway. I've worked hard at it and now I can hit it through a keyhole."

At the conclusion of the clinic, Trevino stopped to wipe sweat off his hands and face, something that surprised me. His swings seemed so unforced, it did not look like exercise. He leaned on his club (again), and gave off that practiced casual air Trevino exudes in public.

"It's the clubface, folks," he said. "The clubface can be square, open, or closed. The ball must always obey the clubface. And who controls the clubface? You do, folks. Learn where your clubface is at all times during the swing."

Someone in the audience asked how to stop slicing the ball.

"You mean like this?" Trevino said, simultaneously hitting a big banana ball that swerved to the right. Several heads nodded, the ball flight so instantly recognizable.

"And when you do that, you instinctively aim more to the left, hoping to balance out the slice, right?" he asked. "What you should do is aim to the right. Aim right where that slice is ending up."

And when he did that, Trevino of course launched a beautiful right-to-left hook. And he got several members of the audience to come out and prove that Trevino's tip was not only logic but physics.

"We've made average golfers think they're dumb, or at least too dumb to figure this game out," Trevino said to me afterward. He was seated in an anteroom off the pro shop, away from a small ballroom full of people who awaited his arrival for a reception.

Trevino, it always surprised me, avoided crowds when he wasn't competing or performing. In private, the Merry Mex is indeed an inapt nickname. He is quiet and restrained and lets others do the talking. He practically refuses to answer the telephone, adopting the attitude of fellow pro Fred Couples, who when asked why he doesn't answer the phone answered, "Because there might be someone on the other end."

But on the subject of what ails the everyday golfer, Trevino could not help but speak up.

"People need to take lessons from a golf pro, but that's because they need to understand the role of certain basics: grip, stance, alignment," he said in a low voice. "But it doesn't have to be rocket science after that. They should experiment with some things like they would in any other sport. The club is in their hands; they can make it work.

"It doesn't take expert analysis. It takes practice. Master it like you would anything else important to you."

I've played golf with Trevino on a few occasions. On a golf course, he is such a people magnet and so universally popular that you get his attention only in small bursts. He may have said he would play with you for nine holes, but he would frequently be tugged away to join this group or that group. Someone would want a picture or to hear a story. Trevino knew the role; he knew how to make people happy.

Still, I remember practically every moment of the few holes I played with him. Not so much because it was thrilling to be playing with Lee Trevino — one of my childhood heroes — but because of how much he taught me.

The sophistication of his golf advice is in its simplicity.

After I hit two out-of-control hooks, he had me grip the club and slapped the back of my left hand hard — twice. It hurt.

"Ouch," I finally said.

"The back of that hand must face the target through impact," Trevino said. "You've got to hold it on through. And if you don't, smack yourself in the back of the hand. Keep hitting it until you remember not to turn over."

Later, I mishit a sand shot that scurried past the hole. Trevino had me get back in the sand with another ball, then he adjusted my stance so the ball was about 18 inches closer to my left foot.

"Put that ball forward and you can swing as hard as you want," he said. "And swinging hard is good."

And on and on this kind of stuff went. It took him less than twenty seconds to give me a tip I could use for the rest of my life: Chip with a 5-iron from 40, 60, or 100 feet off the green if your approach is relatively flat ground; hit from thick rough by pretending that you've got a shovel and are digging a hole; chase down and after the ball with your right shoulder to hit crisp iron shots.

His suggestions were like magic. I would do them and instantly play better.

It is what golf's immortals can do, at times give us the panacea, or at least make us think they have the cure-all remedy. We watch them play, we watch them demonstrate shots, and we believe golf can be simple, and better, it can be fun. We see the evidence in their gifts, in their play, and in their smiles. And I have come to believe that in the end they have never forgotten that this is a game.

One day in the late 1990s Trevino was walking in the eighteenth fairway with me during a media day outing in New Jersey. The sun was out and it was about 85 degrees with a lovely breeze.

"What a day, huh, Bill?" he said.

We were about 100 yards from the green, where I had a 6-foot birdie putt. Despite his tutoring, I had butchered the last two holes (actually, he had been away doing an interview). Now I needed to make this putt if my partner and I were going to win our match. It might even get us the tournament low gross.

"It will be a better day if I make this putt," I said.

Trevino stopped walking. Stopped dead in his tracks and turned to look at me.

"Who cares about that putt!" he said. "Come on, it's a great day. Besides, you'll make that putt."

We took a few more strides up the fairway. He was whistling as we walked. Then Lee Trevino again washed me in his immortal golf god magic potion.

"Just keep your head still and close the toe of the putter a little bit just before impact with the ball," he said. He slapped me on the back, laughed, and walked away, yelling toward the others in our foursome: "What a day, right?"

I closed the toe just before impact and that putt chased toward the hole as if it had no place else to go, disappearing right in the middle.

From the far edge of the green, Trevino did a little dance and pointed his finger at me.

"I told you," he said.

Yes, he did.

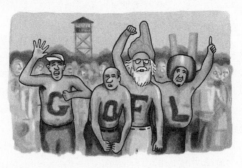

9

Golf Is a Sport; Are You Game?

You can't call golf a sport. You don't run or jump.
You don't shoot, you don't pass. All you have
to do is buy some clothes that don't match.

STEVE SAX, five-time All-Star second baseman

FOR DECADES, THE sporting public — golfers and nongolfers — has been arguing a basic question: Is golf a sport or is golf a game?

It has not been what you would call a good-natured or intellectual argument. To most nongolfers, who tend to view golf with a mix of distrust and bewilderment — as they would a hooded cult setting up tents at the end of the block — golf cannot possibly be a sport.

They look at golfers zipping around on golf carts, swilling beer, and chomping on cigars, and they are not immediately reminded of the physical effort and exertion of a triathlon. A golfer fussily positioning a putter behind a ball, then standing still as a statue — waiting, waiting, waiting — to execute a stroke that might send the ball across the green all of 3 feet does not remind them of the power and precision of a towering 400-foot home run. Watching a golfer casually slipping a wedge through a playful-looking little sand trap does not conjure the image of the courage needed to catch a punt and run it back against an advancing horde of eleven football players bent on knocking you down as fast and as hard as possible.

Admittedly, golf requires skill, but then, so does chess. In that way, the debate goes, golf is more like darts. That makes it a game and not a sport.

Some golfers do not disagree. Some do, and do so vehemently.

These defenders of golf's corporeal honor say that what separates most top golfers from average golfers is indeed an unmatched combination of many essential elements of athleticism: superior hand-eye coordination, the ability to perform a series of movements in sequence and with perfect timing, extraordinary flexibility and balance, mental acuity under pressure, and a hard-to-define but vital dexterity in an unpredictable outdoor environment.

These golfers point to golfer-as-athlete ideals like Dustin Johnson or Camilo Villegas. The other side of the argument points to a puffy, slipshod John Daly or the PGA Tour's Tim Herron, whose nickname is "Lumpy."

It is a frequent barstool debate, and one that can never be settled with a phone call or by checking the almanac behind the bar. There are no *Who Wants to Be a Millionaire* lifelines that will help.

There has been, however, a surprising amount of research done on this subject. Meanwhile, an ever-expanding wing of medical science has been devoted to studying, and fixing, the impact of golf on golfers' bodies. There are such things as golf nutrition and golf fitness. People work at making better use of our senses, like our eyesight, to improve play. Scientists have examined whether being in shape makes you score lower.

Does all this answer the question of whether golf is a sport? See for yourself. A host of people have waded into the debate. I am just trying to quell the arguing so we can get back to important barstool debates, like why nobody calls their 9-iron a niblick anymore. Or why the Professor, if he was so smart, couldn't build a simple raft from the thousands of trees on *Gilligan's Island*.

Dr. Neil Wolkodoff is the director of the Center for Health and Sport Science at the Rose Medical Center in Denver, a book author, and a clinical exercise specialist. As it happens, he likes to settle sports arguments. In fact, it is very nearly his job; every few months he sets up an experiment to test and examine some facet of the ongoing sports continuum. As a golfer, he has been party to the golf-as-sport dispute from time to time. But unlike the rest of us, he has the means to try to ascertain a decisive conclusion.

So a few years ago, Wolkodoff's medical center spent $27,000 on equipment to conduct a painstaking set of tests on amateur golfers. The golfers wore elaborate but portable measurement gear that took periodic readings of oxygen used, carbon dioxide produced, ventilations per minute, and distance and elevation changes. The golfers played the Inverness Golf Club in Englewood, Colorado, a high-quality course that has hosted some top state amateur tournaments. Each golfer played the front nine holes four different times on different days — walking with a pushcart, walking with a caddie, walking and carrying a golf bag, and riding in a golf cart.

Scores were kept and analyzed. Calories burned were counted. Perspiration was measured. Everything was evaluated. The golfers were required to keep the nine holes as standardized as possible. In other words, if they used a driver off the first hole when they played with a caddie, they had to use the driver playing the first hole the other times. Weather was not a factor as each nine was played on similar, somewhat chilly autumn days. The sequencing of how they played the rounds was varied; not everyone played with a golf cart first, then with a caddie, and so on.

Before the experiment began, each golfer went through rigorous testing to establish his aerobic endurance and anaerobic threshold levels — the point when lactic acid buildup generally begins to impair coordination and concentration. This meant that Wolkodoff could watch readouts from six pounds of sensors strapped to the golfers and identify when they had gone beyond their fitness level. That became important because exceeding one's anaerobic threshold quickly went hand-in-hand with ineffective golf.

What Wolkodoff discovered is that playing golf uses more energy than most people suspect. Obviously, the most energy was expended while walking with a bag (721 calories burned for nine holes). But walking with a pushcart was not far behind (718). Walking with a cad-die burned 621 calories for nine holes, and riding in a cart still burned 411 calories on average.

"One of the surprise realizations was that just swinging a golf club about a hundred times uses up a significant amount of energy," Wolkodoff told me.

The golfers walking with a caddie or with their clubs on a pushcart registered the lowest scores. Golfers riding in a cart had the next-low-est scores, and those carrying their own bag did the worst.

What Wolkodoff found most consequential is that golfers who be-came winded or slightly out of breath hit more mishits or had poor outcomes of shots. Think, for example, of someone walking up a steep hill and then having to execute a delicate chip without much rest. This matters because exercise specialists say it can take two minutes to re-store heart and respiratory rates to normal.

We don't usually get two minutes. So being fit cuts strokes.

"If you're out of shape, exceeding your threshold could happen a few times every round, even while riding in a cart, because tee boxes and green complexes are often elevated," Wolkodoff said. "Your golf game will suffer. Somebody missing a short putt might actually just be a little winded after walking up to an elevated green. At the same time, being in better physical condition would make you better mechani-cally and mentally."

Wolkodoff's study, which may be the first of its kind, had its lim-its. Because the equipment was cumbersome and expensive and took about two hours to put on and take off, his test group was just eight golfers. They were men ranging in age from twenty-six to sixty-two with handicaps from 2 to 17.

But it is impressive that the golfers' results during the four rounds tracked similarly with consistent statistical trends. For example, seven of the eight golfers reported the same scoring pattern: lowest score while playing with a pushcart (group average was a 5-over-par 40 for nine holes), followed by playing with a caddie (42), playing with a mo-tor cart (43), and playing while carrying their bag (45).

By the way, Wolkodoff received no commercial sponsorship or fi-nancing for the study other than from the Rose Medical Center.

"It's not a perfect study, but I think we discovered some things," Wolkodoff said. "But if it hasn't been done before, it's because of all the time, equipment, and data involved."

In fact, representatives at the PGA of America, the United States Golf Association, and the National Golf Foundation said they were not aware of studies exactly like Wolkodoff's. A recent University of Pittsburgh study measured one golfer's caloric expenditure as he walked with a bag, walked with a caddie, and rode in a cart. That study put the number of calories burned at higher rates than Wolkodoff's study — about 1,000 calories for nine holes of walking and carrying, 750 for walking with a caddie, and 650 for riding in a cart.

"The health benefits of walking was the best news of our study," said Wolkodoff. "Playing eighteen holes of golf while pushing a cart twice a week shouldn't replace an overall fitness regimen, but it could be a very worthy supplement."

On many golf courses, of course, it isn't possible to walk because golf courses promote the use of carts to raise their revenue. And adding to the popular cart culture is the persistent myth that cart use speeds play even though dozens of studies have proven that to be untrue. Of course, some people cannot walk the golf course for various physical reasons. Still, spreading the word that walking while playing will yield significant health benefits could help the game grow.

"I don't just play golf to lose money to my sandbagging friends," you could tell your spouse. "I do it for both of us because I want to stay in shape."

It would be true, and it would apparently help your score and perhaps your wallet. So in the end, did Wolkodoff answer the burning question: Is golf a sport?

"There are a lot of ways to define a sport," Wolkodoff responded. "But we know that the golf swing uses almost every muscle group in the body. We know it uses a pretty significant amount of energy — not as much as running a 10K but more than people think. And one significant measure of a sport is whether physical training improves your ability to perform, and I think that's been proven in golf.

"So in my estimation, it's absolutely a sport."

• • •

Let's go at this from another angle: If golf isn't a sport, how come so many people get hurt doing it?

I know people get hurt dancing, too; that doesn't make it a sport. But apparently many more people are injured playing golf than dancing. More than 9 million Americans sustain golf-related injuries annually.

What is a golf injury?

Poking yourself with a scorecard pencil? Foot blisters from that sand in your shoe? A sprained ankle from chasing the beverage cart?

"Golf is actually a demanding athletic activity that puts tremendous stress on the body and has a high injury rate," said Dr. Larry Foster, an orthopedist in Carmel, New York, whose book, *Dr. Divot's Guide to Golf Injuries,* details golf-related ailments and how to prevent them. "Golf is a sport. I see the results of the exertion, the competition, and the strain in my office every day."

About 60 percent of players have a golf-specific injury at some point, Foster said, and they can miss from five weeks to a year of activity. It's worth acknowledging and recognizing that statistic, even if you want to keep calling golf a game, because it might help you prevent serious injury.

While a golf injury might sound amusing or inconsequential — a little soreness in your arm, a twinge in the back — it can be as funny as a four-putt on the first green.

"Nobody takes golf injuries seriously until they get one," said Foster, Dr. Divot. "They take it a lot more seriously when they can't tie their shoes because of lower back pain or can't shake hands because of a sore elbow or wrist. Maybe they can't raise their arm above their shoulder or their knee is swollen. Maybe they're having trouble sleeping. It's a big, underappreciated problem."

Dr. Vijay Vad, a sports medicine specialist at the Hospital for Special Surgery in Manhattan, wrote the book *Golf Rx* after he did a clinical study of PGA Tour players with bad backs. Now nearly half of the patients he sees — about 400 to 500 people annually — are golfers.

"People would be shocked to know how common golf injuries are, especially to the back," Vad said. "It comes from overuse, it comes from bad technique, and it comes from a lack of core fitness. The perception that golf is just an easy leisure activity, something you don't need to prepare for like any other athletic activity, is a gross misperception. You need to stretch and prepare yourself for golf as you would for any other physical activity."

Perhaps because the golf swing happens so quickly — less than 1.5 seconds — people think not much is going on. The opposite is actually true. Because it happens so fast, the torque and stress on the body are significant.

In Foster's book, he notes seventy-seven medical studies on the injuries that can occur in those 1.5 seconds.

Among the things that can go wrong, lower back issues are the number one problem. They account for about 35 percent of all golf injuries. Elbow strains — essentially "tennis elbow" in a golfer — account for 33 percent.

Wrist and hand injuries, including fractures, often occur when players abruptly strike the ground or an object during a swing, and they represent 20 percent of the injury total. Shoulder problems (predominantly rotator cuff tears) account for 12 percent. Knee injuries, like tears to the meniscus, are 9 percent of the total.

A vast majority of elbow, wrist, hand, and shoulder injuries are to the lead side of the body in the swing, which would be the left side for a right-handed golfer. Women are just as susceptible to injury as men, although they have fewer back injuries. One theory is that men develop higher club velocity and rely more heavily on forceful trunk rotation during the downswing. In other words, they want to impress their friends with their distance off the tee and swing too hard.

Prevention of golf injuries is not complicated but only because the science of the infirmities has been thoroughly investigated. According to Vad's PGA Tour study, lower back problems might actually be caused by a lack of hip flexibility. Examining pro players, he discovered that those with less flexibility in their lead hip, the left hip in a right-handed golfer, had more back problems than those with limber hips. Here's how that makes sense: You have to swing a driver about 80 to 90 miles per hour, or 110 to 120 miles per hour if you're a pro, and you have to bring that high-speed swing to a stop in a little more than a second. As Vad told me, "Try asking your car to do that."

Various shock absorbers in the body withstand the deceleration forces, but for those who are not very flexible in their hips, the forces tend to go to the lower back. Do it 100 times, or 300 times counting practice swings, and you've got a strained back.

Some golf injuries, like elbow or wrist problems, are caused by flaws in our swings. Not to add insult to injury, but if you are a hacker with a slice, you are more likely to hurt some part of your arm because you probably release your wrists prematurely when you swing. If you start the downswing with your wrists instead of your hips and shoulders, not only will you be looking for that sliced shot in the woods, you might also be trying to rub the tendinitis out of your leading elbow.

Since golfers get as obsessive about their sport (or game) as other athletes (or hobbyists), there is another common cause of injury: overuse. In fact, reaching for the jumbo bucket at the range is usually a bad move unless you hit that many balls every week.

"Unless you hit one hundred balls a day like some pro, going out on a Thursday night and whaling away nonstop for an hour is at the least going to make something sore, which is a mild strain," Foster said. "It also might cause a more debilitating strain or inflammation. As the saying goes, everything in moderation.

"And take some breaks so your body recovers. Mix up the clubs you use so you're not taxing the same groups of muscles over and over in the same way."

The golf docs also want you to try to break a sweat before you play. You might feel ridiculous, but a light jog from the pro shop to the first tee might be good for you and your golf. You could do a few jumping jacks on the practice range beforehand. Or run in place for twenty seconds. When no one is looking, wave your arms in a circular motion to loosen up your shoulders. At the very least, take a brisk walk around the back of the first tee or the clubhouse for a couple of minutes. Whatever you do, don't just sit in the cart waiting for something to happen. What will happen eventually is an injury.

That's because the muscles, tendons, organs, and various other body parts work better with a little internal lubrication and that comes from adequate, or increased, blood flow. So get your blood pressure up just enough to warm up your golf machine. You wouldn't ask a cold car engine to do too much until you had the chance to rev it up a little. The same goes for your golf body. Get it cranked up before you crank it up.

Dr. Foster says a little forethought can go a long way — and make the ball fly longer, too.

"Look, I'm not a good golfer," he said. "If I break 100, that's a good day. So I know how overwhelming it can be. But I tell my patients that if they do the preventive things to engage in this very physically demanding activity, they won't have to see me regularly — unless they see me hacking away on the golf course."

Since a certain amount of golf fitness can prevent some of these golf-specific injuries, Dr. Vad has developed golf-specific exercises to help prevent injury and to add distance to your drives. They can be as simple as lying on your back with your knees bent and feet flat on the floor. Then alternate bringing one knee to your chest. Another begins standing upright, with the feet shoulder-width apart. Twist to touch the fingertips of your right hand to your left ankle. Do the same with the left fingertips to the right ankle. This is an exercise that all golfers could certainly do on the first tee. If you can find time to do them regularly off the golf course, you might be happier still.

"Ten to fifteen minutes of core exercises done two to three days a week can accomplish a lot for your golf swing," Vad said. "Even leaning against a wall and stretching your hamstrings before you play will help. Drinking plenty of fluids can prevent a back injury."

That's because dehydrated muscles are fatigued, which makes them more likely to strain and tear under the stress of a golf swing, Vad said.

Some of the medical prevention advice is very golf-specific. Foster, for instance, worries about golfers who aren't reasonable when their ball comes to rest on a tree root or rock. His recommendation? Move the ball and take the penalty stroke if you must, because trying to hit it is inviting trouble.

"It's great that so many golfers want to play by the rules and do the right thing," Foster said. "But in many cases, is it really worth it? I've had people come in and tell me: 'I hit the rock, broke my club, and I couldn't play the rest of the day.'

"They end up with a wrist so painful they can't play for weeks, can't brush their teeth with their dominant hand, and can't hold a fork with it either."

When Foster asks them why they didn't just move the ball, they often respond that they were playing a match with friends. For $5 a side. Now, I ask you: Would a game make you that crazy? Or would it have to be a sport?

If golf is a sport — we're leaning in that direction, right? — then it must require training. And Neil Wolkodoff's experiment seemed to prove that fitness can lower your golf score. In twenty-first-century America, there is no more booming, compulsive movement than the desire to be fit and healthy. Perhaps it is not surprising, then, that a small army of kinesiologists, fitness gurus, and golf nutritionists have descended on the golf community to help golfers to the promised land of golf fitness and well-being. Golf fitness has become a cottage industry.

One of the best-known golf fitness gurus is Katherine Roberts, who appears on the Golf Channel to demonstrate exercises. She has written several books on the topic as well. When I met Katherine years ago, I told her I didn't need to improve my golf fitness because I still worked out. I ran fifteen miles a week. She told me, nicely, that I didn't know what I was talking about.

"I hear that all the time," said Roberts, who is a trainer and yoga instructor. "Golfers say, 'I'm in golf shape; I walk forty-five minutes a day on the treadmill.' And I'm glad to hear that people are doing something active. But they're not training for golf, and before too long, they're probably not going to have the flexibility and strength to play as well as they want to — or used to."

Roberts then asked me a few (leading) questions. Like whether there was a hole on my home course — like a par 5 — that I used to sometimes reach in two. She asked if there were any milestone features on the course that I used to mark my drives by.

And come to think of it, there was that sprawling oak on the uphill par 5 that had been the measuring stick for a drive long enough to go for the green in two. I hadn't been reaching it much lately, usually by 15 yards or more. And the tulip tree next to the dogleg on the third hole, the one I always hooked my drive around to get past the bend? I was usually 10 yards short of that now.

"Why do you think that is?" she asked.

I had just figured that someone moved those trees farther away.

Roberts wasn't convinced. She had another theory.

"Some loss of flexibility, maybe a little less core stability," she said. "Maybe you need to be in better golf shape."

Katherine prescribed a golf fitness program to integrate into my normal workouts. It focused on enhancing the flexibility in my hips, back, and shoulders, while also adding strength to my core to improve my balance. Living in New York State, I am geographically challenged for winter golf, so I did Roberts's exercises over my off-season. It added about forty-five minutes to my exercise regimen for the week. It also helped me regain the length and, perhaps more important, the consistency I had lost. It's amazing what restoring a little suppleness to your frame will do. I am not promising booming drives of 275 yards, a gratuitous goal anyway, and certainly not what I achieved, but even a simple program can help far more than you may think. And most important, it will help more golfers play the sport (snuck that in) longer and enjoy it more.

Here are a few exercise examples Roberts recommended, from her book *Swing Flaws and Fitness Fixes,* which she wrote with Tiger Woods's former coach Hank Haney.

The most practical exercise is called the Plank: Having a well-conditioned core is critical to the dynamic phase of the swing. The plank position strengthens your abdominal muscles. Place your hands directly under your shoulders, squeeze your legs together, and keep your back straight. Hold for thirty seconds to a minute and repeat three times.

Another exercise is called the spinal-hip-hamstring series. With an elastic strap around your right foot, extend your left leg. Press your left hip toward the floor and extend your left arm perpendicular to your body. Hold for five breaths. Extend your right leg to the right, maintaining the connection between your left glute and the floor. Place the strap in your left hand and bring your right leg and hip to the left.

The third exercise is called a revolving shoulder twist from a lunge:

Bring your left knee forward to a lunge position. Bring your right hand to your left knee. Hold for five breaths and switch sides. For more of a challenge, put your right elbow on your left knee, your left hand on top of your right, and turn your right shoulder away from your ear.

Roberts, not surprisingly, is not the only one who understands the value of simple, understated golf workouts.

"A golf fitness regimen starts out as something you do to lower your score," said Dr. Greg Rose, a cofounder of the Titleist Performance Institute, a golf fitness center in Oceanside, California. "People aren't thinking about their health at all. But it ends up making you more fit overall. It recharges people. And they play better."

Added Dr. Vad: "We're all living longer and people don't want to retire and sit on the couch. They know the importance of aerobic exercise, but unless they tune up their musculoskeletal system, things often break down playing something like golf. So then they will play less, be in more pain afterward, and score higher, too."

There are a lot of ways to get started with a golf-specific exercise program. The Internet is awash in suggested drills. There are numerous books. Roberts in her book identifies particular swing faults — like the reverse pivot — and provides exercises aimed at attacking that imperfection. Dr. Vad's book promotes a fifteen-minutes-a-day program.

At the Titleist Performance Institute, touring professionals receive high-tech physical and club-fitting assessments. Amateurs can also receive the star treatment with a visit costing from $5,000 to $10,000. But Rose and other experts at the institute have traveled the world to certify more than 3,000 golf, fitness, and medical professionals in the institute's training methods. They have certified pros across the United States and in dozens of other countries. Their Web site (www.mytpi.com) has a system for finding therapists, trainers, golf pros, and chiropractors who will evaluate you and your golf swing and devise a routine of exercises aimed at your problems, be they tight hamstrings, inflexible hips, or a weak shoulder. The cost for this initial assessment is about $125 to $300. You can receive personal attention for the workouts at the certified centers as well. And the institute's Web site has a vast array of golf fitness articles and videos to help customize a program.

"What matters is that people understand that even fifteen or thirty minutes four times a week will reap tremendous benefits," Roberts said. "It's about doing it with regularity. A short, simple program done four times a week works far better than a two-hour workout once a week.

"You don't even need to go to a gym," she said. "But if you sit around all winter watching football and your only exercise is shoveling the driveway, you're not giving yourself much of a chance to be physically prepared or more physically equipped when golf season resumes."

But then, isn't that a given for many of us? A lot of golfers know they aren't very good and don't believe a little stretching and strengthening are going to make them any better. Sure, PGA Tour pros work out ninety minutes every day. So does my cousin Jerry, and he can't hit a golf ball 200 yards, let alone 320.

"The game frustrates most golfers, but when you give them a physical exam and tell them that their lead hip or an unstable shoulder is what's holding them back, they light up," Rose said. "It gives them an excuse for what's been going wrong, and they no longer think it's all their fault. They have something to work on. It gives them hope."

And there is no golf without hope.

If the expanding assembly of fitness gurus and kinesiologists are concerned with the outward manifestation of your golf swing and all its moving parts, then the smaller cadre of golf nutritionists are trying to convince you that what you eat and drink can greatly influence the flight of your golf ball.

At face value, this might not prove golf is a sport, but it does contribute to the substantially important notion that golf is a demanding physical and mental activity that cannot be performed at a high level without a prepared body. And apparently, not without a well-nourished one either.

Plus, it's interesting and cool to think that some nuts swallowed on the front nine will keep you from going nuts on the back nine. There are all kinds of cause-and-effect nutritional equations.

Is a slice driving you mad? That banana ball off the tee may be cured with a mid-round banana. (I told you bananas were underrated.)

Topping the ball? Perhaps you should have topped that morning bagel with peanut butter. A fried egg might have seemed like a good breakfast, but it could be causing those fried-egg lies in bunkers.

Now, you may think this is tofu-eating mumbo-jumbo. If you're faltering in matches, it's because you have the yips over 3-foot putts. But nutritionists would have an answer for that as well: Low blood sugar from poor food choices can cause nervousness. You are what you eat, they say, or at least consume, and in golf it may be truer than you think.

How about this: Do you have guys at your club who take beta blockers for high blood pressure? Doesn't that give them an edge in tense, stressful matches? Beta blockers are also antianxiety drugs — musicians, opera singers, and other performers often take them to quell stage fright.

Some of the drugs intended to treat attention deficit disorder help people without the condition to concentrate and focus. They, too, could help golfers. The professional golf tours think so. They have begun testing the players for these drugs.

In Germany last year, twenty golfers spent six weeks eating energy bars with 200 milligrams of phosphatidylserine, an ingredient linked to better concentration and coordination. During this period, when measured against a control group of golfers with similar handicaps who did not consume the energy bar, the golfers plied with phosphatidylserine began to hit their tee shots noticeably closer on a 148-yard par-3 hole, according to researchers conducting the study.

Now, we can take this too far. I do not think that golfers losing matches or tournaments across the land will soon be gathered in nineteenth holes muttering, "I've got to double my phosphatidylserine intake next week."

At the same time, with golf rounds increasingly lasting four and a half to five hours, and with the touring pros having proved that fitness and overall good health help produce lower scores, it makes sense that we could fuel ourselves a little better.

Dan Benardot, an associate professor in kinesiology and health at Georgia State University and the codirector of the Laboratory for Elite Athletic Performance, has some suggestions. He recommends that someone preparing for a 9:00 a.m. match might want to get up a little earlier to finish eating breakfast at least ninety minutes before playing. Benardot suggested a glass of juice and some toast, something amounting to 400 calories. Another nutritionist, Nancy Clark, recommended the bagel with peanut butter, or cereal and nuts.

"An earlier meal will stabilize you, and you'll need the boost it brings," Clark said. "Golf may not be marathon running, but it does require repeated, high-intensity swings that are coordinated, athletic movements like in other sports."

Note, she said *sports*. The key, the nutritionists said, is not to avoid calories in this active setting. They recommended consuming enough carbohydrates to sustain proper blood sugar levels during play. Benardot said golfers should be sipping a sports beverage throughout their round — maybe a few mouthfuls every other hole. There are many beverages in this category made by Powerade, Gatorade, and Power Bar. Some have golf-specific concoctions. They all will work just fine.

Clark, the author of the *Sports Nutrition Guidebook* — key word: *sports* — said she would have golfers take granola, energy bars, or trail mix to eat on the course. Clif Bars are portable and very filling. There are golf energy bars called 1st Tee and 10th Tee.

And what of the typical mid-round golf choices, the standard hot dog and beer?

"If you're having a social round of golf, maybe that's OK, but if you want to play well, those are completely nonsensical choices," Benardot said. "Throw the hot dog away and eat the bun; that has carbohydrates."

I guess Slim Jims and Jell-O shots are out of the question.

Well, like everything else in golf, it's about course management. I wondered, though, what real effects I would see in golfers who did not seek the recommended nourishment.

"They would get irritable, jumpy, nervous, and cranky," Benardot answered.

Actually, that sounds like my regular foursome.

The point is that there are time-honored, traditional food choices at the golf course — egg-and-cheese sandwiches for the early risers, hot dogs and sausages at the turn, beer, soda, chips, and candy from the beverage cart. A lot of it is not good for you or for your golf. Maybe we shouldn't treat a visit to the golf course like it's a visit to Uncle Leo's poker game. Remember, golf is a sport, not a game. This is golf, not five-card stud.

As with almost any sport, the role that our sense of sight plays in performance cannot be undervalued. It is no different with golf. Does this prove anything? It does if you realize how much what we see, or don't see, can affect our golf. It is an overlooked part of succeeding at golf. The eyes control more than you think.

Several years ago, Joan Vickers, a researcher at the University of Calgary, discovered that elite putters had what she termed "quiet eyes." These players kept their eyes absolutely still for a few seconds before and after striking a putt. Less accomplished putters moved their eyes rapidly, darting from target to ball and other places on the green.

Dr. Mark Guadagnoli, a golf research scientist at the University of Nevada–Las Vegas who works with top amateur and professional players, described a correlation between eye movement and brain activity. "A quieter eye also quiets the brain," he said. "You can teach someone fairly quickly a technique to quiet their eyes. We have done it in our lab."

He suggested that golfers standing over a putt focus on a spot behind the ball, instead of on the ball itself. One goal is to eliminate sensory intrusions from the task at hand. Guadagnoli has players say "da" on the backstroke and "da" again to complete the stroke, which serves several purposes, including giving the golfer something to ponder besides the usual negatives like "I hope I don't miss this easy putt."

Also, research has shown that when most putters focus on the ball, the brain instinctively wants to track the ball after it is hit. Hence, the dreaded head lift while putting. Focusing on a spot behind the ball, Guadagnoli said, makes the brain, and eyes, less likely to follow the ball.

"The quiet eye works in the full swing, too," said Chris Bertram, a professor of kinesiology at the University of the Fraser Valley in British Columbia. "We've studied golfers with goggles that measure eye movement, and the more skilled ones lock on a specific target ahead of them and then focus entirely on the back of the ball. The lesser players have jumpy eyes — one look at the green, one look at a pond, then they look at their club, then their feet, the ground. Their eyes are still moving in that critical one second before they start their swing."

Now, tell me that doesn't sound just like the average duffer. Here's where I would expect my eyes to be focused over a testy shot — one look at the green, one look at a pond, another look at the pond, especially to notice that the ripples are still on the water from where my previous ball landed, one look at my club, another look at my club because I'm wondering if it's a 6-iron or a 9-iron (I've made that mistake before), one look at my feet, another look at my feet because I've noticed that I haven't shined my golf shoes in eighteen months, one look at my grip on the club, another look at the grip because I don't think the Vs of my thumbs and palm are pointing at my shoulders like I heard they should be last night on the Golf Channel, another look at my grip because I notice that my glove has mustard on it (I thought I licked that off), one look at the ground, except I can't see the ground because I'm in so much high rough I feel like I'm standing in a cornfield, one look on the horizon for the beverage cart because that reminded me that I'd really love some corn Cheetos . . .

So basically, I don't have quiet eyes. But I should. As Dr. Guadagnoli explained, taking the eyes out of the full swing can help, too. Guadagnoli has had golfers close their eyes when hitting balls on the range.

"We can become too reliant on our eyes, which is our most dominant sense," he said. "You'd be surprised how much you can tell about a shot, and eventually your swing, by listening to the sound at contact and judging the shot by what you feel happened."

Guadagnoli told a story about a nearsighted golfing partner who could not see shots past 200 yards "but always hit the ball straight, so it didn't matter."

Then Guadagnoli's friend had Lasik surgery and soon started hitting more wayward drives. "My theory is that he started turning his head to watch the ball," Guadagnoli said.

Now, that's pretty freaky.

Could anything this complicated, this convoluting, and this contradictory be only a game? Could something that tests our anaerobic thresholds, our musculoskeletal structure, our metabolic production, and everything else from our hip flexors to our eyesight — all in the quest to put a ball in a hole — could that be anything other than sport?

Well, it could be a waste of time, too, but you think that only when you shoot twenty strokes higher than normal.

But seriously, if you are still on the fence about whether golf is a sport, know this: Whatever golf is, it ought to be played and played often because golf is good for you. It may even save your life. For this you do not have to take my word.

According to a study of 300,000 golfers in Sweden, golfers live longer than nongolfers by about five years. This was true for golfers regardless of sex, race, or occupation. Leaders of the study said the health advantages were linked to players' being outside in fresh air for several hours and walking briskly between shots. More amazing: The data showed that golfers with the lowest handicaps lived the longest. Researchers reasoned that because golf is good for you, playing it more often (typical behavior for better golfers) yields even more benefit.

I rest my case. No mere game can do all that.

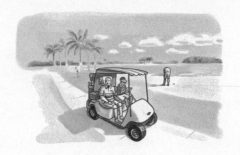

10

Golf Safety

> If I'm on the course and lightning starts, I get inside fast.
> If God wants to play through, let him.
>
> BOB HOPE

I HAVEN'T SAID too much negative about golf in this book, because, well, there's nothing negative to say. Who doesn't love golf, right?

But some golfers can love it too much. And it can lead to trouble.

As I've said many times already, golf is good for you — for the exercise, the fresh air, and the socialization benefits. Heck, doing the math as you try to keep track of all the side bets is good stimulus for the brain. But we can get too much of a good thing, and I'm not talking about hand calluses or back spasms. Some harmful extremes lurk on the golf course.

I'm not trying to scare anyone, and I'm certainly not advocating we play less golf. (We all want to live five years longer like the golfing Swedes.) But like many things in life, advances in medicine and science have made it plain that some common habits are not good for us. Consider some of the things we used to do off the golf course. About half of the population used to smoke, people believed exercise in adulthood was bad for your heart, and they thought salads were for rabbits. Over time, we have learned differently.

It should be the same in golf.

For decades, there have been very few health and wellness admonitions when it comes to golf. Golfers were warned not to stand in front of someone else when they were hitting, a rather obvious warning that still goes unheeded. Golfers were told to be careful looking for lost balls near seaside cliffs — another "duh" moment. If you were playing a desert course, you were told not to chase errant shots into the sand and scrub unless you really liked snakes.

I've played in Canada and Montana where I was reminded that moose roam the fairways and it is best not to try to hit them off the tee because an enraged moose can run forty miles an hour (faster than a golf cart).

Ponds were not considered dangerous, but the large and often ornery snapping turtles that sun themselves near the ponds can be. Don't get too feisty with the geese or swans near those water hazards either. If their young are around, they will chase you. I don't think they could really do you any harm, but you will be the source of relentless mockery for the rest of the day — if not the year — should your partners see you sprinting in fear from a waddling, livid goose flapping its wings.

(Larry David in an episode of *Curb Your Enthusiasm* killed a prized black swan in this situation. Suffice it to say, it did not turn out well.)

Other than those perils — most of them wildlife-related — golfers were told to have at it. Go enjoy yourself in the large, green outdoor playground of golf.

And you should. The dangers are few and controllable.

But just as there is now room in most of our diets for salads — and even vegetables — there is room in our golf bag of sensible behaviors for a dose of prevention and an understanding of what can go wrong out there.

Two golf hazards, for example, not discussed nearly enough would be the danger of lightning and the risk of skin cancer from the sun.

If you play enough golf, you are regularly exposed to both.

In a typical year, lightning kills more people than tornadoes or hurricanes. A golf course is an especially threatening place during a thunderstorm because it has isolated, tall trees and wide-open spaces where golfers can be the tallest target. Dermatologists, meanwhile, say golfers are notoriously poor at protecting themselves from sun damage and frequently need treatment for harmful lesions on ears, hands, and noses.

And as much as it may seem obvious to avoid golf balls struck by other golfers, people do get hit by shots regularly. Serious injuries occur, and there are definitely ways to minimize that risk. Then there is the golf cart, a seemingly harmless little aid to the golf community. Except when it isn't. The golf cart, it turns out, is another overlooked hazard. Apparently, it should come with a siren and flashing police lights.

Of course, the first, most dramatic threat: lightning. Anyone who spends long periods of time outdoors is susceptible to a lightning strike, and golfers are especially vulnerable because we have a code that seems to honor persevering in tough weather conditions. Once out on the golf course, we don't want to leave it. There are all kinds of funny sayings about the fanatically devoted golfer, little jokes about how we won't come off the golf course.

"It never rains on the golf course," people say.

"Nae wind, nae rain, nae golf," the Scots say.

And golfers everywhere like to declare that "a terrible day on the golf course is still better than a good day at work."

Lee Trevino certainly never feared he would be struck by lightning.

"I lived in Texas where lightning rose up quick in the sky, left quick, and we never thought too much of it," he said.

Then in 1975, Trevino was struck by lightning while playing in the PGA Tour's Western Open. He sustained injuries to his spine and had surgery to repair damaged discs but was hampered by back problems for years thereafter.

"And when it happened, it wasn't even raining," Trevino said. "Just *boom!* It wasn't a direct hit but it came up through the ground and got me."

Two-time United States Open winner Retief Goosen was fifteen years old and playing golf with his friend Henri Potgieter at the Pie-tersburg Golf Club in South Africa. A slight drizzle began to fall when lightning suddenly struck the ground near the boys. Potgieter was knocked off his feet, and when he stood back up, he saw Retief mo-tionless on his back.

Retief's clothes had burned off, his watchband had melted into his wrist, and his shoes had disintegrated. His tongue was back in his throat and he was hardly breathing.

"I remember picking up his spectacles and I didn't know what to do," Potgieter told the magazine *Golf World* years later. "I thought he was dead and I started screaming for help. Fortunately, there were guys teeing off on the next hole and they came running. They picked him up and put him in a car."

Retief Goosen recovered fully although he still has a scar on his wrist from the incident. He could not wear shoes for weeks. He did resume playing golf eventually. And like most touring pros, if he hears thunder, he leaves the golf course — regardless of how much money is on the line.

Several years ago, while covering the Westchester Classic tourna-ment outside New York City, I was one of twenty-five or so writers the pro golfer Rocco Mediate called together for a lightning awareness seminar. Mediate had never been struck by lightning, but he knew of golfing friends who had been seriously affected, and he began working with the National Weather Service to educate golfers.

With Mediate that day was Michael Utley, a recreational golfer from eastern Massachusetts who was struck by lightning while playing on Cape Cod.

"I don't remember what happened; I didn't remember anything for thirty-eight days after I was struck," Utley said. "But my friends who were with me said they heard the loudest noise they had ever heard, and when they looked around I was smoking and falling to the ground. Luckily, one of my friends had recently taken a CPR refresher course and he started reviving me.

"My heart stopped several times and I was revived several times but I made it to the hospital. About thirty-eight days later, I was feeling well enough to start the rest of my life although I had lost all learned memory. I had to relearn all the basic functions — walking, eating, dressing myself.

"One day I was just a guy worried about whether I could get to the green with a 7-iron. Then everything changed."

Utley smiled as he told the story and he seemed healthy and fit again. But he added: "I wish somebody had told me more about lightning risks like I am telling you now."

This kind of thing happens often. A few years ago on a driving range in Colorado, a lightning storm passed through with dozens of golfers hastily seeking shelter in their cars. Thinking the storm had passed, most went back to hitting balls. Then, nineteen golfers were knocked out and hospitalized, with the lightning passing in an arc from golfer to golfer on the range. All survived, although some were left with permanent injuries.

Golfers being struck by lightning when they come back too soon is common, and lightning experts say you should wait thirty minutes from the last time you saw lightning. But even more common are golfers who are struck because they don't leave the golf course when they see lightning in the distance or hear some distant rumble of thunder.

Golf is addictive and hard to walk away from. And sometimes we think, "But I'm playing so well today," or "It took me two months to get this tee time."

I know I have done that. But I don't do it anymore, in part because I attended the presentation by Mediate and Utley. And because of conversations I've had with lightning researchers like John Jensenius.

Jensenius has for years investigated every injury caused by lightning in the United States from his office at the National Weather Service. He interviews all the victims, if they survive. And when it comes to golfers, he said many had advance warning because they heard thunder in the distance.

"The golf course is one of those places you can usually see a storm coming," Jensenius said. "But a lot of golfers don't head in, thinking they have not yet seen lightning.

"Unfortunately, every thunderstorm has its first flash of lightning, and that one is as deadly as all the others," Jensenius said.

Lightning often strikes ten miles from any rainfall and can strike ahead of storms or seemingly after they have passed. Jensenius said golfers should examine the sky and plan.

"On a golf course, if you hear any thunder, you should head inside a building or a hard-topped car as soon as you can get there," Jensenius said. "I study the case histories of all lightning fatalities. Often, if people had gotten inside five or ten minutes earlier, they would be alive. All the cases are very sad; these are good people who make a mistake."

Jensenius said golf clubs and other metal objects do not attract lightning. This is a persistent myth that lightning experts work hard to debunk, with limited success so far in most quarters. The fact is, experts say that lightning occurs on too large a scale to be influenced by small objects on the ground whether they are metal or not. Lightning bolts can be several miles long and may emanate from a cloud eight miles above the ground. That lightning bolt is heading down from perhaps 50,000 feet, so it is not influenced by your 3-foot-long metal clubs, or your metal jewelry.

Another myth: The rubber tires in the golf cart will protect you because they ground the vehicle. Even in a car, it is not the rubber tires that are offering the protection against lightning. Jensenius said getting in the golf cart will offer little shield from the dangers of a lightning strike. As for the rubber tires misunderstanding, no one in the lightning safety community knows where that got started. It seems sensible but it's not true. In fact, unfortunately, farmers rank high in the catalog of lightning victims. They are hit riding tractors — with rubber tires. Many lightning victims are struck riding lawn mowers with rubber tires. Cars are safe, lightning experts say, because they have metal roofs and sides.

As for those huts you sometimes see on the golf course, the ones that you probably thought would protect you from lightning?

"They will probably only protect you from rain," Jensenius said. "There isn't anywhere on a golf course that's safe unless it's a sturdy structure built to withstand a lightning strike. That means it has walls."

A maintenance building or shed with electricity might do the trick but not a wooden portico.

The National Weather Service offers safety guidelines and suggestions online at www.lightningsafety.noaa.gov. A few other sobering facts: The majority of lightning victims are children or men younger than forty, which suggests to Jensenius that behavior or peer pressure plays a significant factor in who gets struck. About 85 percent of victims are men.

"Being safe is inconvenient," he said. "I'll add that most people struck by lightning do not die, but most are left with lifelong neurological problems."

The debilitating symptoms include memory loss, sleep disorders, chronic pain, numbness, stiffness in joints, muscle spasms, and depression.

"I know golf is a great sport," Jensenius said. "But it will be a great sport after the lightning has passed."

And after you have waited another thirty minutes.

Unlike lightning, which strikes quickly, the danger golfers face from exposure to the sun comes in opposite form — it accrues over a long period of time. But even casual golfers spend hundreds if not thousands of hours in the sun over a lifetime. We love to play, and since golf is such an absorbing task, our mind can easily be distracted from the beating our skin takes on an unrelentingly hot day.

And some golfers don't really get sunburned, or they have skin that appears to have adapted to the sun. In each case, damage to the skin can still be occurring. Other golfers rationalize that they are not really in the sun that often since they are riding in a golf cart. They are forgetting how long it can take four golfers to chip onto a green and putt out. Or how much time is spent waiting to hit on the tee box.

Golfers are highly susceptible to skin cancers brought on by overexposure to the sun.

The Women's Dermatologic Society for several consecutive years has conducted free skin cancer screenings at select LPGA Tour events across the nation, with doctors examining fans, caddies, and volunteers.

"About 45 percent of the people we see at those screenings have something on them that's going to have to be treated, and that's a much higher incidence rate than the general populace," Dr. Marta Rendon, a south Florida dermatologist who has participated in about a dozen of the golf tournament screenings, said. "We see skin cancers and a lot of precancerous spots. The screenings have saved a lot of lives."

For some reason, perhaps because women are more conscious of their skin than men, LPGA players take the steps to protect themselves from the sun far more than the male professionals. Walking with LPGA players Christina Kim and Paula Creamer at a pro-am tournament one year, I was struck by how often they applied sunscreen.

"We've lost some caddies to skin cancer out here and something like that really shakes people," said Kim. "They were one of us. So we've been more aware of it for a while, but I can tell you that we talk about it more now than ever. There's always sunscreen in our lockers at every event, and we'll remind each other sometimes. You know, at the turn, 'Hey, more sunscreen every nine holes, girl.'

"It's on people's minds. It's amazing to think how people used to play golf for hours without putting any protection on their skin."

Dr. Wendy Roberts, the president of the dermatologic society, has her practice in Rancho Mirage, California, a Palm Springs Valley community known for its many golf courses. She said specific problem areas for golfers include the back of the hand not usually inside a golf glove and the lips, which should be protected by balm with sunblock.

"Men also completely forget about their ears, and they miss the patch of skin on the side of their neck just below the ear," Roberts said. "I remove a lot of cancers from that spot."

She added: "I have golfers tell me that they're being careful because they wear a hat or a visor, but when I ask if they put sunscreen on their legs, they say they didn't think of that because they're in the golf cart a lot. But the leg is the number one site for melanoma in a woman and number two in men."

The LPGA has a sun-safety initiative, and many of its players preach the sun-protection gospel. The Women's Dermatologic Society has been a partner with the help of a grant from L'Oréal USA and has created a Web site with golf sun-safety tips, www.playsafeinthesun.org. One tip that has stayed with me is the lesson of reapplying sunscreen every nine holes. If you think about it, if you were exercising on a beach for five straight hours, would you apply sunscreen just once?

Tom Kite, the 1992 United States Open winner and native Texan, learned he had skin cancer in his fifties. He blames the culture he grew up in, where a golfer's tan was a badge of honor and a sunburn was just a minor inconvenience for getting to play golf.

"When I was a kid, you weren't even considered a real man unless you lost the skin on your nose three or four times a summer," Kite told me once. "I've adopted a new attitude and all golfers should."

Kite wears a wide-brimmed hat outdoors and applies sunscreen to his arms, hands, and neck.

"A golfer has to remember that we're busy on the golf course," Kite said. "We're trying to make shots, trying to win matches, or just trying to get a few extra yards out of our driver. Our mind is preoccupied. So we don't remember every minute we're in the sun.

"But our skin does."

Chances are, from the beginning of golf, golfers have been hitting other golfers once they wind up and swing. We all know the golf ball seems to have a mind of its own sometimes. We can smack a driver 250 yards down the middle and then five minutes later, hit the ball 25 yards sideways. We can hit it backward. I have seen people hit themselves with their own shots. You can snap hook one off your shin or spank it off the hosel so that it bounces directly between your legs and then ricochets straight up.

Ouch, that hurts.

Reminds me of an old golf joke. Golfer coming off the course to his friend: "I hit only two good balls all day. Yeah, stepped on a rake."

Anyway, the bigger danger is getting hit by another golfer's errant shot. And there are precautions that both the swinging golfer and the watching golfer should take. The first step is realizing you are both responsible for making sure no one gets hurt.

If you have a golf club in your hands, you should be making sure your playing partners are a safe distance from you. I know they are crazy enough to play golf with you and that might make them unpredictable knuckleheads, but before you swing, try to find each playing partner so you know they are not in harm's way.

The next most important thing you can do is be very mindful of where everyone is during your practice swings. In the handful of times I have seen someone injured on the golf course, half of those injuries have not involved the ball at all. Someone got hit by a practice swing instead. People on the tee box are often inattentive and not altogether mindful of what's going on around them. And they tend to wander around. Once people address the ball they put their guard up, but be very watchful of your group on a crowded tee. It's not the best place to swing your driver four times as you try to develop tempo. If you must do that, go to the back of the tee or get off the tee entirely and do it far from the group.

When it is your turn to hit, don't swing unless the group in front of you is completely out of range. Avoid the temptation to hit the ball as they are moving out of range because you have been waiting ten minutes and are frustrated by the pace of play. Better to cool off and wait. You won't likely hit it well if you have any doubt in your mind that the hole is clear in front of you.

When it is not your turn to hit, plan for the highly unexpected. This is golf; the highly unexpected happens all the time. So don't stand 10 yards in front of another swinging golfer even if you are 30 yards to the right or left.

Have you not seen shots that travel 30 yards to the right and 10 yards forward? You probably have seen that in the last hour.

Don't tempt golf fate. Stand back from and off to the side of other golfers whenever you can. And watch their shots. It is courteous to help track the ball, and if you're watching, you might just have time to duck when they hit it backward/sideways.

Another way that golfers get injured on the golf course is in the pursuit of an off-line shot that went into an adjoining fairway. Don't walk or ride into the other fairway without checking to make sure golfers playing that hole aren't teeing off or about to launch a shot in your direction.

If you should hit a shot so crooked that it might strike someone ahead of you or someone on another hole, yell "Fore" as loud as you can. And should you be the one who hears the yell of "Fore," for goodness' sake don't turn in the direction of that admonition to see where the ball is. That's a good way to get one in the face.

What you want to do is make yourself smaller. Crouch, turn away, and cover your head with your arms. All golfers should be familiar with the fetal position anyway. Golf will leave you that way sooner or later.

The last topic in my guide to safer golf concerns a most overlooked piece of risky golf equipment and that is the golf cart. It is not a dangerous vehicle in the hands of a reasonable driver, but there is something about a golf course that suspends people's natural prudence and turns them into a gaggle of Evel Knievels. Golfers tend to drive the golf cart as if it were on tracks, like something at an amusement park where nothing can go wrong.

Golf carts do look like fun and we treat them like playthings. Admit it, when you were nine years old and your mom or dad asked you if you wanted to play golf, your first thought was "I might get to drive the golf cart."

But it is amazing, and a little scary, all the crazy things people do with golf carts. In my regular Google alert for the word *golf,* I have come across some astonishing mischief, mayhem, and misfortune that ensue when people get behind the wheel of a golf cart.

For one, people dump carts in golf course ponds with stupendous regularity, and they submerge them deep enough that the police and heavy-duty tow trucks have to be summoned. One golfer outside San Jose, California, nearly drowned when he tried to swim to shore with his golf bag around his neck. I bet there was a brand-new melonheaded driver in that bag. Or a dozen Pro V1s. (You can also insert your own joke about a melon-headed cart driver here.)

But seriously, you have to ask yourself, isn't it pretty hard to dunk a golf cart in a pond? I can see losing a ball in a pond. I can see losing ten balls in a pond, even on one hole. But a cart? I've never seen a cart path that leads into a pond. Can you really be so distracted by how badly you're playing that you don't see the water coming up before the green?

The other thing people do in golf carts is drive directly into lowhanging tree limbs. That causes some head injuries. They hang their feet out the side of carts, too, which leads to a lot of broken ankles when a limb is twisted by a landscaping element, like a greenside railroad tie or a flower bucket. People fall out of golf carts as well, and rolling a golf cart is not uncommon.

The golf cart itself seems to have contraptions that, when mixed with golf, lead to problems. Not long ago, Erik Johnson, once the first overall pick of the National Hockey League draft and a pivotal player for the St. Louis Blues, missed an entire season when he tore the anterior cruciate ligament in his right knee at the team's annual preseason golf outing. Johnson got his foot stuck between the accelerator and the brake of a cart and tore up his knee. A year later, Matt McChesney, a reserve offensive lineman for the Denver Broncos, stepped out of his golf cart just as another cart zoomed past him and struck him in his recently rebuilt ankle. The injury ended up forcing the twenty-eight-year-old McChensey to retire from football without playing another game.

Some pro teams have clauses written into contracts prohibiting players from golfing during the season. I always thought that was because they didn't want players baking in the sun for five hours before a night game. It turns out it may be to keep them away from the golf carts.

It kind of makes sense in a weird golf sort of way that something as innocuous as the golf cart with its cushy seats, floppy, oversized tires, and extra handy straps becomes the very thing you have to fear the most — not the spiky shoes, rock-hard golf balls, 47-inch weighted drivers, or pointed tees.

The Center for Injury Research and Policy at Nationwide Children's Hospital in Columbus, Ohio, studied golf cart injuries and reported in 2010 that nearly 148,000 golf cart–related injuries occurred between 1990 and 2008. The number of cart-related injuries rose to nearly 13,500 in 2008, from about 5,700 in 1990. So we're getting worse as golf cart drivers, not better. These injuries were not sustained exclusively at golf courses, but a large percentage were.

"A lot of people are getting hurt because they do things in a golf cart they wouldn't think of doing in an automobile," said Dr. Lara McKenzie, one of the authors of the study. "People on the golf course are having fun, and that's good. But the golf cart is a motorized vehicle that can go fairly fast. And children fall out of them because they are built differently than adults, and without a seat belt, they don't have the balance or the strength to handle some bumps or turns."

The doctor had additional safety recommendations: Keep your feet flat on the cart floor, avoid sudden turns, use the hand grip above your head for stability, and don't make any post-factory changes to the cart, like disabling the speed governor.

There is, of course, another way to handle this situation: Hire a caddie.

A caddie might also be able to warn you should you be standing too near another golfer getting ready to hit. A caddie might remind you to use your sunscreen. And a caddie might definitely seek shelter if a thunderstorm was approaching.

All caddies know that the most important, overarching objective of a day of golf is to live, and stay able-bodied, to play golf another day.

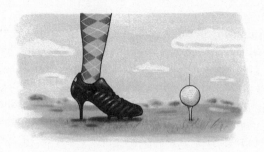

11

The New Culture of Golf

Fantasy, Fashion, Finance, and the Forsaken Golf Ball

The only time my prayers are never answered
is on the golf course.

BILLY GRAHAM

Not to generalize, but people who take part in fantasy sports leagues are obsessed lunatics.

Unless we're talking about fantasy golf leagues. Because they're OK.

A lot has changed in golf, and in the modern version there are many new accouterments affixed to a ritualized, tradition-bound game. Golfers were once a staid lot who dressed alike — and poorly at that. Golfers were traditionalists who did not swiftly adopt or accede to new trends. A contemporary golfer was one who no longer wore knickers and was willing to try one of those newfangled metal drivers — which in a classic case of golf contrarianism they still referred to as a "metal wood."

But look how far we have come. Golfers have now waded into the great sea of unwashed fantasy sports players. But wait a minute. We aren't really lumped in with all of those crazies, are we?

No, of course not. Fantasy golf is the restrained, distant cousin of the other unmannerly, imaginary fantasy sports. In golf, for example, the annual player draft is a cordial affair, in a room filled with guys wearing polo shirts speaking in hushed tones. Our imaginary teams are full of gentlemen playing a game of decorum and integrity.

Perhaps that's why my young son has taken to calling Sundays in the spring and summer "the afternoons when Daddy screams at TV golf for two hours."

So I admit I am a fantasy fraud. I acknowledge that fantasy golf makes me, and many other participants, an obsessed lunatic. Indeed, we may be worse than players of other fantasy sports, and here's why: Not only do we let golf humiliate us on the course, but we also go home and watch another golfer on television, chosen as our representative, as he or she is humiliated by this faithless game as well.

Fantasy golf leagues are not nearly as big as those operated for professional football or baseball, which have combined to lure more than 30 million people into an addictive stew of stats and strategy. But because fantasy golf has far simpler rules that require little number crunching, its popularity is growing rapidly. More than 6 million people now participate, according to Peter Schoenke, the president of Rotowire.com, a site dedicated to fantasy sports.

In fantasy golf, you can be a math simpleton and not feel as if you will be outwitted by the accountants and actuaries in the competition. Try that in a fantasy baseball league. The United States Congress wanted to rewrite the IRS tax code a couple of years ago but realized all the top mathematical minds were too busy with fantasy baseball.

But golf fantasy leagues are easy and welcoming. For example, I belong to a fantasy golf league of a dozen friends. Once a year, each of us picks a team of ten golfers. The champion is the owner whose ten players cumulatively amass the most PGA Tour money. Simple as a 3-foot putt to win the match, right?

Some leagues require players to pick a different golfer, or three different golfers, every week. Some follow only the major championships. There is a league in which you win by picking the worst golfers, those who record the highest scores.

Now, that is cruel, and genius.

Yahoo, PGA.com, CBS Sports, and several other Web sites run fantasy golf leagues. They can be free, although some have small fees ($25) and relatively small first-place prizes ($500). In higher-stakes leagues, the fee can run $300 and the payout $5,000. The basic reason fantasy golf exists, though, is to enhance interest in an otherwise bland tournament as you're sitting in front of the TV on a Sunday afternoon — in other words, when none of the big-name golfers are in contention.

But if fantasy golf's rules are simple, its culture is not. Having a team means worrying about things other fantasy sports players never have to consider. If you are in an NFL fantasy league, your players may have injuries, but you never have to worry that Peyton Manning will decide to sit out a third of the Indianapolis Colts season because his wife is pregnant. And Aaron Rodgers is not likely to take off the first two weeks of October because his girlfriend breaks up with him.

Pro golfers, being the self-employed businessmen they are, do these kinds of things all the time. They also sit out tournaments to attend their kids' birthday parties. When that happens, I can hear a nation of fantasy players yelling: "Hey, Vijay, back away from the birthday cake and get your golf bag to the Greater Milwaukee Open. This party is costing me money!"

So picking a fantasy team means knowing every detail of a golfer's personal life. The prototype for a fantasy golf magazine would read like a gossip weekly, dishing on who's going out with whom, who is distracted with the building of a new $10 million house, and who is too busy adding to his 10,000-bottle wine cellar to visit the practice putting green. Or stagger to it.

The skinny on drinking habits would be key. Golfers have a lot of free time.

A fantasy golf magazine would also have an entire section devoted to the pros' vacation plans.

You think I'm kidding? I guess, unlike me, you didn't draft Chris DiMarco for your fantasy golf team in 2006, when he was ranked in the top ten worldwide. A week after our draft, he went skiing with his kids, fell, and cracked some ribs. He hasn't been the same since.

You also didn't have Ernie Els the year before, when he blew out his knee riding an inner tube with his kids during a Mediterranean vacation. One stray wave ruined my whole year.

And don't even get me started on Sergio Garcia, the talented boy wonder I took with my first pick in 2009. That was the year Greg Norman's daughter dumped him. Shortly thereafter, Garcia told a British tabloid that she was his first love and he has been in a funk since. Did I mention that Garcia, formerly ranked number 2 worldwide, essentially took the rest of the year off and fell out of the top one hundred on the PGA money list?

So this fantasy golf business gets complicated. Still, it does bring a lot of exhilaration to the common, calm Sunday afternoon.

Several years before I had been lured into this dark world, I was in a country club grill room on a Sunday when over in the corner, a guy was yelling at the TV — "Miss it! Miss it! Miss it!" — as the little-known Joey Sindelar lined up a short putt to win the 2004 Wachovia Championship.

"Wow," I thought at the time, "how could anybody hate Joey Sindelar that much?"

Nowadays, that scene wouldn't faze me at all. I would understand that the guy glued to that TV had a fantasy golf team and that one of his players was a stroke behind Sindelar.

Been there, done that.

Except I usually yell a little louder at the TV.

Golf Fashion

Nothing has changed as much in golf's new world order as what golfers wear on the golf course. Raise your hand if you have heard of Sansabelt. Step to the front if you know what it means. OK, go back to the rear of the room; some of you are still wearing your Sansabelt pants. That's enough of that.

Sansabelt pants were big among golfers — and other groovy guys — in the 1970s. They were trousers that had a wide elastic band sewn into the waist, which was intended to make a belt or suspenders unnecessary. Get it? Sans a belt?

They were trippin' rad, hip, funkadelic, and they let you keep on truckin' all the way to your crash pad. Jack Nicklaus wore Sansabelt pants, as did Johnny Miller and Tom Watson. Just about every regular golfer in America had at least one pair of Sansabelt pants. You could play eighteen holes in the afternoon and not even have to change before you headed to the disco. You would, however, have to change your shoes. For one, they had metal spikes then, which wouldn't be safe on the dance floor when you were doing those John Travolta leg splits, and two, the shoes had foolish-looking lace flaps and tassels. They looked a little like something a four-year-old beauty pageant contestant would wear. Elton John might have worn them in concert.

The average golf shirt then also had long, pointy collars that drooped down to the armpits. You know that practice drill where you put a golf towel under your right arm and keep it there to keep your elbow from flying out on the backswing? In the 1970s, guys just tucked their collar under their arm.

Golf socks, meanwhile, were louder than a drunken conventioneer. Belts were as wide as an eight-track tape and just as pliable. Golf hats were so pointy they made everyone look like a relative of the Coneheads.

Oh, and did I mention that the Sansabelt pants had 18-inch-wide bell bottoms that caught in the rough and dragged in the goose droppings?

Yes, it was a natty, refined game back then.

And to think this was supposed to be an improvement on the days when golfers wore tweed coats and ties. Give me the professor garb before the pimp look, any day.

Women golfers, meanwhile, did not have it much better. Luckily, they were generally pushed toward more conservative garb and more of them wore shorts. But essentially women's golf fashion was men's fashion in smaller sizes. At least they didn't have to wear the Conehead hats.

All these years later, have things improved? Well, except for Ian Poulter and his Union Jack pants and shoes, yes, they have.

In fact, most recreational golfers I know are envious of pro golfers and how they dress. The pros look great in their golf clothes — far better than average golfers look. How do they do that? Everything matches perfectly, even the belts and hats. Everything looks crisply tailored. They don't look like regular golfers at all. The collars aren't rumpled and the shirts don't sag at the belly.

Let me tell you a little secret. Top golf pros don't put together those combinations. They have clothes picked out for them in advance like a kindergartener. When it comes to a major championship, the clothing has been selected and assigned to each golfer nearly a year in advance. A small army has been at work to make them look sharp.

Here's how it works:

For the top players, it is called "outfit scripting," and it includes the color and design of the shirt, pants, and hat for all four rounds. It usually includes the footwear, although some players are finicky about their shoes. All the major golf apparel manufacturers — Nike, Adidas, Ashworth — do it for each of the four majors championships and most regular Tour events, too. They dress their golfers like walking storefront mannequins. It's all a marketing ploy. They decide months ahead of time what a Tiger Woods or Luke Donald will wear on the final day of the Masters so they can be sure to have that exact outfit on store shelves the next day.

"A single shirt worn by one of our athletes on a Sunday afternoon winning a tournament can raise sales 10 percent," said Tiss Dahan, the senior director of global apparel at Adidas Golf. "We see the influx online, and our customer service phone line will get the calls from retailers who are reacting to requests from consumers. They want the shirt, belt, or hat they saw on TV. You get somebody playing well in clothes that look good, it really moves the needle for apparel."

If you think that's an exaggeration, consider that golf apparel is a $4 billion business in the United States. Consider also that the winner of a major golf tournament could be on television throughout the world for five consecutive hours. His or her face and clothes will appear on Web sites and in newspapers, and the winning outfit could surface again a month or a year later on magazine covers.

So to make the most of this opportunity, the scripting process begins for most companies with a design meeting about a year and a half before an event. New looks in stripes, plaids, and prints are examined, as well as the technology of materials, such as moisture-wicking fabrics. A color palette is chosen and a decision made on how the basic clothes will work with vests or pullovers. The golfers are consulted regularly. Tiger Woods, for example, meets with Nike's apparel team three to four times a year. In the last of those meetings, he is shown prototype garments for his approval or rejection.

"Tiger won't wear green pants, for example," said Doug Reed, Nike's global director of golf apparel and accessories. "One year, we proposed he wear a dark green shirt on a Saturday at the PGA Championship. Tiger took one look at it and said: 'The PGA is in Oklahoma in August. There's no way I'm wearing a dark shirt in that heat.' So we took it out of the script."

Various pros have their own preferences. For a long time, Mike Weir would wear only black shoes. Anthony Kim and Rickie Fowler like to be daring, hence the bright spangled AK belts and orange-from-head-to-toe Fowler outfits. Others are conservative, like Justin Leonard and Davis Love III. And, of course, no two players should ever arrive at the course in the same outfit. A few years ago at the U.S. Open, there was consternation on the first tee when Phil Mickelson's caddie arrived in the same shirt as the golfer Charles Howell III, who was playing in Mickelson's group.

Mickelson, by the way, for a few years had no clothing contract. He picked out his own clothes with the help of a London tailor. Shocker! His clothing was widely panned by the golf fashion intelligentsia. They hated his propensity for white belts because they felt the belts called attention to his not-so-svelte torso. They despised the button-down-collar look he sported, noting that only men with long, slender necks should wear tight, button-down collars — and Mickelson's neck was judged too compact.

And you thought you were just watching a golf tournament on TV.

The companies script clothing for women as well, although not as precisely. "We can send the female golfers a box of clothes and they put them together very nicely," Dahan said. "They often choose exactly what we would have chosen. For the top women players we have exact scripts but we don't get too technical. We don't devote as much time to it as to the men."

Two reasons for that: Women's apparel is only 30 percent of the overall golf apparel market, and industry experts believe women recreational golfers are more likely to mix and match to create their own outfits, so TV scripting is not as important.

For all the planning, male golfers sometimes go off the script because they decide to wear a lucky hat or shoes from the day before. So a green hat ends up matched with a red shirt and white pants. The designers turn on the television and cringe. Green, red, and white? It's not even Christmas season.

"You have moments when you want to cover your eyes," Reed said. He said he has the same reaction sometimes when he sees everyday golfers.

"Average golfers could learn a lot about how to dress on the golf course from studying the pros," Reed said. Other designers echoed that sentiment. When pressed, they gave me a few simple recommendations for how the weekend golfer could be a little more fashionable:

Men should consider buying at least two pairs of quality golf pants. Many male golfers have none. The number one reason pro golfers look better than regular golfers is their choice of superior fabrics and blends. The pants that pros wear are usually a worsted wool or high-grade polyester blend. You can buy the same kinds of pants; you just have to step away from the rack of cotton khakis. And they will cost you maybe twice as much.

You may not want to spend $80 on a pair of golf pants, but here's why it's often worth it. Quality fabrics are more durable, fit better, and hold their shape longer. You should have a couple of pairs of higher-quality golf pants for those occasions when you have to play in a special member-guest or when you get invited to play golf with the boss. For the price of a dozen Pro V1s you will look considerably more put-together. Let's say the pants last fifty rounds. That's an extra 80 cents a round.

Also, find the shirt fabric that makes you most comfortable. For decades in golf, that fabric was cotton. And that still may be your personal choice but not necessarily your best one. Golf shirts have gone high-tech with moisture-wicking properties, antiwrinkle systems, and intricate synthetic knits. So don't just grab the same polo. Most pros now wear more sophisticated blends, and they are not generally more expensive.

As Eddie Fadel, the vice president of Ashworth Golf, said: "It's pretty easy to find a golf shirt that will still look good after you've worn it a dozen times because of the engineering that has gone into golf wear. We don't want recreational golfers walking around in our stuff and have it look shabby or out of sorts. That's our logo on the shirt. If it doesn't look good, other people won't want to buy it. That's our best advertising, a garment that looks good on you."

You don't have to be a fashionista. Just pay attention to the makeup of your golf shirt. It's not 1990 anymore.

Next, pay attention to at least one underappreciated accessory. The belt you wear to mow the lawn is probably not a good choice for the golf course. You don't have to spring for a $175 Italian leather golf belt, but there are plenty of reasonable options from $20 to $50. You could buy one $28 black belt and one $28 brown belt and probably cover all your options for years.

For advice on women's golf fashion, I went to two of the top female names in the game. Paula Creamer suggested that women be more experimental than they might in their everyday wear.

"It's the chance to go a little wild with more bright colors," she said. "Get away from the black and khaki look." Nonetheless, Creamer stressed functionality and shorts, skorts, or pants with "lots of pockets."

"They always make men's pants and shorts with lots of pockets because you need them for tees, ball markers, and other things," Creamer said. "But they used to avoid pockets on women's shorts to make them more stylish. But there's a way to do both. You can hide the pockets."

Morgan Pressel, consistently ranked in the top twenty worldwide, said women should shop for their golf clothes in golf shops as well as department stores.

"I think the idea is to get your basics, your golf clothing staples, in the department stores," Pressel said. "But you're going to want a special outfit or two. You need to go to a golf specialty shop for that. And there are plenty of them. That is where you will find shirts or shorts with special features. That's where you'll be able to put together a nice, eye-catching combination: top, bottom, and hat. Or, a woman might find a nice golf dress. There are a lot more of them than ever — and they have pockets now, too.

"These are the kinds of things that make a difference to a woman and it will be worth it to her. Most golf shops nowadays do a good job providing women with variety. We don't have to look like women wearing men's clothes in smaller sizes."

Taking this advice is probably a good idea because it's safe to say that you won't have anybody scripting your golf wear, which is probably a good thing. Not many of us want to look as if someone else picked out our clothes anyway. But you don't want to show up at the first tee looking like you just found your shirt rolled into a ball in your golf bag and decided to wear it anyway.

And don't laugh; you've done that. I've seen you on the first tee.

It might also be a good idea to have shorts or pants lacking motor oil stains. I know you don't play golf for the fashion possibilities. You want to put together a run of birdies at the local muni, not put together an ensemble for the Milan runway.

But it isn't hard to look presentable. It will make you feel better and, yes, probably even make you play better. Knowing you look the part is one less thing to worry about as you prepare for that first shot of the day.

Remember, though, no button-down shirts if your neck is too short.

Golf Finance

Golf, people like to say, has always been a moneyed sport. It's more stereotypically true as a cultural touchstone than a reality. Just because a lot of rich people play golf it doesn't mean all people who play golf are rich. The opposite is actually true. How do I know this?

Well, the average round of golf in America costs a little more than $20. If you exclude the East Coast and the highly populated areas of California, the average golf round is only $14.

Wealthy people playing golf on exclusive golf courses represent a minor, almost tiny, slice of the golfing public. Their game is not our game. (Just as their annual $20,000 country club dues are not, thankfully, the same as the $30 we pay annually for a county resident card and its golf course discounts.) Now, I'm not saying that people do not spend significant sums of money on the golf course. They do. It is just paid out in small increments.

More than ever, the new golf culture is one of extra dollars thrown here and there. The economic future of golf as baby boomers continue to retire is probably tied to all the new revenue streams golf courses can invent to pull more dollars from golfers' pockets. The possibilities are limitless (fortunately so is my maniacal golfer's imagination).

I've been thinking about this ever since 2010 when California governor Arnold Schwarzenegger wanted to impose a 10 percent state tax on the price of a round of golf. Taxing golfers who endlessly pursue a little white ball around a wide-open field seemed a bit like taxing dogs for chasing their tails. Schwarzenegger's proposal was roundly criticized and voted down, but I found it offensive for other reasons. It was a gross underestimation of how much money could be made off the common, overwhelmed golfer.

Let me take you, for instance, to the first tee, where all you need is an attendant and a cash register:

A mulligan? That will be $1.

What? Another one? That's $2.

Permission to reposition the tee markers, which are devilishly aiming everyone toward the woods? Another dollar.

Completely overcome with first-tee jitters? For $5, the assistant pro will hit your first shot for you.

You get the idea. Charities sometimes do things like this at golf outings, but my golf tariffs would be a public service to the game. The goodwill tax could start as soon as you arrive at the course. Toll lanes could be built on the approach to the clubhouse, like those on highways. For an extra $10 when you are late, you get the express lane with a high-speed bag drop, where they shove you in a cart, change your shoes, remove the fifteenth club cluttering your bag, wipe your face with sunblock, and whisk you to the first hole.

If you're a frequent, on-time customer, you get the $5 prepaid E-Z Pass lane. This leads to a drive-through window on the side of the pro shop, where you can buy golf balls, a glove, and tees. It funnels to an HOV lane leading to the practice range.

The range itself could be layered with services. For $3, you get a bucket of balls and a place to hit off a rubber mat. For $5, you get to stand on a grass surface. For $7, you get a spot in the no-talking section, where no one may loudly and persistently explain the intricacies of some miracle swing tip recently learned on the Golf Channel.

For $10, you can warm up in the business golf/CEO sector of the range, where someone younger will stand behind you as you hit balls and repeat various phrases, such as:

"Your swing has such rhythm and balance; it's so athletic."

"That's a beautiful, practiced draw" or fade.

"Wow, you crushed that one; have you been working out?"

"I hope someday I can play golf like you."

You see where this is going, right? I envision cash register kiosks all over the course.

Let's say you hit your ball in deep rough off the fairway. For $5, a maintenance crew member could choose this exact moment to trim the grass in the area near your ball. He was going to mow there sooner or later anyway.

For another $5, the worker could accidentally run over your opponent's ball with the tractor.

In terms of gear, there is no reason golf carts must be so minimally equipped. They ought to come with hotel-minibar-type vending machines. Beyond alcohol, they could be stocked with antacids ($5) and antianxiety drugs ($20).

Golf courses could start charging $1 for pencils with the scorecard. Better yet, they could charge $5 for pencils with erasers, the ultimate golf tool.

There ought to be computer monitors hanging from the roofs of carts. For $10, you could search the Internet for tips to fix things that are going wrong in your game. Playing a big match? For $25, you could arrange to have the computer in your opponent's golf cart play a stream of golf-tip videos. That ought to ruin his or her game.

It wouldn't harm any golf course to have an official club-throwing station once every nine holes.

Say you've just dumped three balls in the pond fronting a tough, long par 5. Wouldn't you pay $5 at that moment to go to a designated club-throwing area, where an attendant could give you some old wooden driver to safely fling into an unoccupied field? There would be a line for that. For $20, they would let you dead lift an entire bag of clubs and heave it.

On another hole, golf courses could set up a Dr. Phil Whine Center. For a fee, you could sit down for sixty seconds with a psychologist and complain about how unfair golf is.

"I swear, the last time out I shot an 80 and never missed a fairway. I'm a good golfer; you've got to believe me. What's happening today is just ridiculous and not really me. . . . Why? Why?"

You would pay $5 for that. Your playing partners would pay $20 if it meant they didn't have to listen to you.

There could also be an all-encompassing, anti-cell-phone charge of $10 at the start of every round. This would pay for trained attack dogs, positioned at every hole, to charge anyone pulling a cell phone from his or her pocket. It's not as hazardous as it sounds; the dogs would stop chasing you when you dropped the phone. Then they would mash the phone to pieces with their teeth.

Who wouldn't pay to see that?

Golf courses could have an illegal ball hole every nine holes. This is where, for $5, you are allowed to pull out the rock-hard illegitimate extra-distance ball that you bought on the Internet and let it fly off the tee. Or you could use something like the Polara ball, a ball with an asymmetrical dimple pattern that reduces slices and hooks by 75 percent. The ball almost always flies straight.

It is nonconforming to the USGA rules. For $5, you get to pretend you don't know what USGA stands for.

In fact, why not have a "No Rules of Any Kind" hole every nine holes? There could be a guy dressed in a blue blazer with a special "Rules Official" armband waiting at the tee. For $20 per foursome, your group would get to blindfold the Rules official, spin him around five times, and shove him in the direction of a shallow pond.

From there, you get to play the hole however you like. Want to spray cooking oil on the driver clubface before you hit? Go ahead. (The reduced friction can add 25 percent to a drive's distance.) Want to throw the ball out of a deep bunker? Sure, why not throw two balls to see which one gets closer? Want to tee it up in the rough? Perfectly accepted. You don't want to get grass stains on your grooves. Everybody on the green automatically one-putts? Why not? It could have happened anyway.

Just be polite. When you're done with the No Rules hole, have somebody take the cart back to the tee to help the Rules official wring the pond water out of his socks and pat dry his blazer.

For another $20, you would be allowed to slip the rule book out of his vest and tear out page 77, which governs Rule 25-3 (what to do if you hit a ball onto the wrong putting green). Nobody, even Rules officials, has memorized that rule.

But that is cruel.

The point is, there is plenty of money out there to be had, and as golf evolves in a society growing increasingly accustomed to making incremental automatic payments for things, the golf course as we know it will progress with it. I have come up with some inventive extremes in the last few pages, but in a serious way, could golf ball dispensers on many tees be far away?

Why hasn't somebody thought of that? Or a smartphone app for each golf course where the club pro describes the hole you are about to play and relates advice on where to hit your tee shot?

Golf courses already allow groups to text food and drink requests; what's to stop them from allowing you to message the pro shop to request a new driver to demo for the rest of the round for $20? Or a new putter for $10?

Why should you suffer the rest of the day with a club that is ruining your round? It would be against the Rules to change equipment like that, but in many a friendly foursome, would anyone really care?

What price do you put on the collective morale?

There is plenty of money available out there if golf courses do not undervalue the foibles, the vulnerabilities, and the eccentricities of golfers. And I don't think golfers would notice these little add-on costs. We are already paying for a lifetime of torment.

The Forsaken Golf Ball (the Life and Times of the Modern Lost Golf Ball)

Once upon a time, golf balls were made of relatively soft materials, and the average golf ball after being struck a few hundred times would almost split in half, or begin to unravel. If you found a lost golf ball in the woods and it had been there more than a couple of months, it would be nearly decomposed. The balls would dissolve in time in water, and sometimes the cover of the ball would fly off on contact. It was as if it imploded. If your golf ball landed on a cart path, it would get a dent that turned the sphere into a strange globe with a small flat side. Try hitting that ball straight.

The modern golf ball is nothing like golf balls made even fifteen years ago. Today's golf balls are made of different, almost indestructible polymers that do not rot away. They are hard to cut. They are resistant to water (even if seemingly attracted to it). If they strike a cart path, they suffer no more than a little scratch. They fly farther and straighter and keep their color longer. Modern golf balls last forever.

That's a good thing. Unless you lose one. But you're not going to lose one, are you?

The impact and destiny of the modern, but lost, golf ball has almost become a celebrity cause in contemporary golf. Not just for where they go — and they go everywhere — but for the fact that they keep coming back. The lost and newly recycled golf ball is a global, lucrative business and a fascinating, if peculiar, window into golf as it is played.

Who cares about a lost golf ball? You would be surprised. Lost golf balls are easily ignored, until you realize just how many of them there are.

For instance, in a 2010 sonar search for the Loch Ness monster, scientists with a submersible device instead discovered more than 100,000 golf balls.

Who knew the Loch Ness monster even played golf?

In a logical conclusion, Scottish officials surmised that golfers along Loch Ness had been using its twenty-one square miles as an oversize driving range. As a local lawmaker said, "Golf balls are humanity's litter in the most inaccessible locations."

No one knows precisely how many golf balls are lost each year worldwide, though the total in the United States is estimated at 300 million. The worldwide estimate exceeds a billion annually. Hundreds of thousands of golf balls are lost or abandoned every day in lakes, ponds, forests, wetlands, deserts, backyards, gardens, parking lots, cemeteries, on rooftops, and at the bottom of woodchuck holes.

But in the last few years, the simple, seemingly inconsequential lost golf ball has stumbled upon a new international renown and import. Some people worry about the ecological impact just as golf yearns to be viewed as more green. And the arts have discovered the lost golf ball, too. Examining the fate and destiny of the wayward golf shot has been the subject of not one but two glossy coffee-table books.

The lost golf ball, in its own way, has become a fatalistic metaphor not just for golf, but perhaps for life: We are all lost, waiting to be found.

"For every lost ball, there was a forlorn search, perfunctory or thorough," John Updike wrote in the foreword to *Lost Balls,* a 2005 golf book. "These questing ghosts haunt the course, hovering at the juncture of their interrupted game. 'Found it!' one wants to cry out in triumph, though the loser has been decades in his grave."

There has been no recognized study of what has happened or will happen to the millions, if not billions, of lost golf balls dotting the Earth in little white, orange, and pink orbs. There is no accepted wisdom on how long it takes a modern golf ball to decompose in soil or waterways, according to interviews I've done with more than a dozen golf industry and environmental researchers. The informed guess is that most balls begin to break down somewhere between 50 and 500 years. Whether the great multitude of lost golf balls decaying under logs or slowly dissolving at the bottom of swampy estuaries pose an environment hazard is also apparently undetermined. Most scientists seem to think it is unlikely.

Robert Weiss, a professor of polymer engineering at the University of Akron who has conducted extensive research on multipart products like golf balls, said that the zinc in a golf ball is present as an ion strongly bound to the compound. It would not be displaced by water or much anything else besides a sophisticated saw in a laboratory. Weiss conceded that an acid could displace the zinc in the ball but doubted that any waterway is acidic enough to do so.

Weiss did not want to dismiss environmental concerns, but he made what he called worst-case scenario calculations involving a million golf balls in Loch Ness that lost all of their zinc. He estimated that dumping five bottles (ten pounds) of antiseptic mouthwash would deposit more zinc ions into Loch Ness than a million golf balls.

Now, if you are really worried about ruining the planet by playing golf, there are biodegradable, water-soluble golf balls available, though they are primarily one-use balls bought by cruise ship operators so that guests can practice their swings next to the Lido Deck. There are golf balls that are 100 percent recyclable and made from renewable materials. They work just fine but don't fly as far or as straight, and they are hard to get. You won't find them at a neighborhood Target or the local pro shop.

A couple of years ago, the University of Maine started making biodegradable golf balls out of lobster shells. I'm not kidding. And you can play with them, too. Personally, I would be suspicious of a lobster shell golf ball if I were playing an ocean course. What are the realistic chances of that ball clearing an ocean chasm on a par 3? Wouldn't the lure of the salty sea be too much for the lobster ball?

At the same time, I bet if you had some drawn butter in your golf cart — and made sure the lobster balls could see it — you could get those balls to do whatever you asked. Or else.

With so many lost balls lying somewhere, and with the cost of a new golf ball ranging from 75 cents to $4, it didn't take entrepreneurs long to realize the worth of this buried or displaced treasure. There are thousands of lost-golf-ball-retrieval businesses in America. They are hard at work wherever golfers are spraying their shots hither and yon. It is a vast industry, valued at about $200 million annually. Some of these golf ball bounty hunters are teenagers or grammar-school-age kids who wade into ponds after school to find and resell balls at 50 cents apiece.

It can be scary work. I once hung out with two friends, Jimmy Lantz and Greg Siwek, who went into business together collecting golf balls seven days a week on courses in southern Florida. Diving into waterways, they routinely wrestled with alligators, pushed aside underwater snakes and eels, and lost fingertips to snapping turtles in search of golf balls. In eight hours they might find 10,000 golf balls, even as they sparred with the hidden wildlife and climbed over submerged golf carts and ditched cars — all the while dodging errant golf shots, not to mention thrown golf clubs. Each diver lugged a satchel laden with up to 1,000 balls, an air tank, and another thirty pounds of scuba gear that kept them weighted to the pond floor.

Why do this?

It's part of the new economic model for golf. Golf balls are white gold. Lantz and Siwek made more than $100,000 a year reselling their found/lost golf balls.

"People like to tell me I don't have a real job," Siwek, who was thirty-six at the time, told me. "Then I tell them how much I make and their jaws drop."

Lantz and Siwek paid the golf courses a straight fee to work in the water hazards. Before they arrived, they would examine a course map like mining prospectors. They headed to any pond positioned to catch a sliced shot. They often found balls lined up row after row.

"The first time I did it, I couldn't believe how many golf balls were just sitting there all lined up," said Lantz. "It was like playing Pac-Man; you suck up all those little white dots."

They also picked up hundreds of golf clubs, entire bags of clubs, and watches that had flown off players' wrists in mid-swing. In some places, abandoned cars were common, too. "Down in Miami," Lantz said, "the water is like a parking lot down there."

Frequently, the divers were called by club pros or people who lived on golf courses asking if they could look for something specific.

"A guy called me and said his golf bag was in the pond behind his house," Lantz said. "I asked him how a whole bag got in there and he said, 'Well, me and the wife were arguing.'

"Then there's always the guys who want us to look for their watches. They always say they lost a Rolex, but we've never found one. What we find is a Timex or a Seiko."

One of the days I was with Lantz and Siwek, they came upon a 4-foot alligator at a course in Boca Raton. The alligator surfaced, seeming to play at the water's edge with the bubbles that the divers' air tanks had produced. But when Lantz and Siwek — heads down as they scooped up balls — got closer to the alligator, the animal swam in the other direction.

"He's a little guy and a little afraid," Siwek said, laughing. "They get a lot more frisky in mating season."

Later that day, Lantz and Siwek took a break and struck up a conversation with a passing foursome. When it came time to dive back into the pond, Siwek handed the golfers eight ultrawhite balls from his satchel. When one of the group remarked that giving away the harvest was no way to run a business, Lantz asked, "Well, what are you going to do with those balls, fellas?"

"We'll start hitting them," the golfer said.

Lantz answered: "Then they'll be back. We'll get them next week."

I remember at one point I told them it seemed like hard, dangerous work.

"You're right," Siwek said. "Let's be serious, not everybody looks at a murky, slimy, alligator-infested pond filled with golf course pesticide and fertilizer runoff and sees a business opportunity. But we did. It's not necessarily something you can do for too long. It's not a career."

I called Siwek eighteen months later — hey, always stay in touch with a good resource for quality used balls — and he had left the golf-ball-retrieval business.

"I had to get out of those dark ponds," he said.

At the other end of the spectrum is someone like Gary Shienfield, whose Toronto-area company sells more than 20 million reclaimed golf balls a year.

"People don't like to pay $40 a dozen for golf balls," Shienfield, who has partnerships with 2,200 golf courses to recover lost balls, said. "Instead, they come to us on the Internet for that ball at $20 a dozen. They are preowned golf balls. They probably bought a preowned BMW, too."

Also driving Shienfield's profits are sales to India, Vietnam, and much of Southeast Asia.

"Those countries are really taking to golf and they want value, but they also want brand names," Shienfield said. "We ship them anywhere and get plenty more ready."

Like my Florida diving buddies, he understood this new piece of golf's evolving economy.

"We don't sell balls," he said. "We rent them."

Charles Lindsay wrote the book *Lost Balls*, and his second volume, in 2010, more or less on the same subject, was *Bad Lies*.

"Golf is a shared experience and so is losing a ball," Lindsay told me. "One of the great universal things about the game is that even the world's best players lose golf balls.

"Every lost golf ball was once a shot of hope and aspiration that then became a plop in the water."

Lindsay, who has become something of an expert in lost golf balls, said he laughed when he read the reports of 100,000 golf balls in Loch Ness. Having wandered upon hundreds of golf balls in difficult-to-reach places around the world, he did not seem surprised, or worried.

"I doubt they would have bothered the Loch Ness monster," he said. "What would you expect? It's Scotland."

Now, when it comes to lost balls, there is considerable myth and many an argument about whether a lost golf ball that is found and put back in play will perform as well as a new one. There is no definitive answer, other than to say that if it has been lost or submerged in water for more than a year, it will not perform the same. How do you know how long it has been lost?

Used golf balls don't come stamped with a purchase date, but it's safe to say that if it is yellowed or the white covering is faded, it was lost for quite a while. Ball-retrieval entrepreneurs use solutions that whiten and clean up a golf ball, and they are extremely effective. If they can't get it to look decent, it's not going to play decently, that's for sure.

Dean Snell, senior director of research and development at Taylor-

Made Golf, said that a ball submerged in a pond for a few weeks would absorb enough water to lose up to five miles an hour of velocity and would fly a shorter distance. It might also lose some of its spin and launch performance.

Sheinfield, who said his balls are in the water for no more than two or three weeks, lists independent testing results on the company Web site. "For average golfers and the better-than-average golfers," he said, "there is little difference."

About five years ago, *Golf Digest* magazine did its own testing and discovered that top-shelf used balls flew about 6 yards shorter than new ones of the same model when struck with a driver attached to a robot swinging identically every time. Of course, if we could all swing like that, we could break 80 with a gutta-percha.

Sometimes I hear people say that old golf balls, even if they have never been taken out of the box, will not perform as well simply because they are, well, old. Can time ruin a ball's worth?

"No," John Spitzer, the United States Golf Association's assistant technical director, told me. "We've kept them five years and tested them and they are the same as new."

But that's if the balls are stored in a relatively dry place in normal temperatures. Don't buy two dozen golf balls and leave them in the trunk of your car all summer waiting to use them. Don't leave them even for a week if you can help it.

"Excessively high temperatures will harm the performance of a golf ball," Spitzer said. "Bring them in the house. Put them in the den."

Perhaps if you open the box and perch them on a table where they can watch professional golf on television, they will yearn to perform like the balls seen soaring through the sky on the PGA Tour. I have heard of golfers doing stranger things to shave a few strokes off their handicap.

In my house, of course, that wouldn't work. My golf balls would be terrorized by all the yelling at the TV during golf broadcasts. Damn, fantasy golf team.

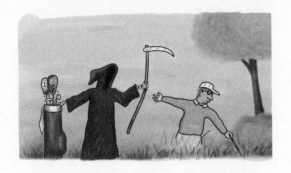

12

Shanks, Choking, and Other Tales of the Dark Side

(What to Do and How to Think When Everything Is Going Wrong)

I'm not saying my golf game went bad, but if
I grew tomatoes, they'd come up sliced.

MILLER BARBER, winner of forty pro tournaments

ABOUT TEN YEARS ago, I played golf at one of those select, fashionable Rocky Mountain resort courses west of Denver. It was a semiprivate club that let tourists on the course on weekdays to raise revenue for a membership that took over on the weekend.

Stealing a day in the midst of a business trip/vacation, I teed off in the early afternoon. It wasn't busy on the course and I breezed through the front nine, which was carved out of an old horse ranch on a valley floor. The second nine, however, meandered through the overlooking hills, which put in play several steep elevation changes. Mountain golf is a treasured experience — the air is crisp, there is always a lot of wildlife around, and the views from the elevated tees are usually majestic and sweeping. Plus, the ball always seems to fly farther (more on that later).

Playing by myself, I was also posting an unusually good score. Most shots were straight and true. The putts were rolling in. Sometimes being alone makes golf easier because you hit your shots at whatever pace suits you. It's also easy to play fast — a single playing reasonably well moves along at a good clip.

I looked at my watch and realized I would probably be done well before 6:00 p.m. when I had told my wife to pick me up at the club. She was off hiking and exploring the area.

On the fifteenth tee, I came upon two guys who had been playing in front of me. I had tried to avoid rushing them from behind, but now as I drove my cart to the elevated tee, I arrived before they had teed off on the hole. They smiled and encouraged me to play through. I offered to play with them.

"No, we've been watching you play; you're too good for us," one of them said. "We're just kind of hacking it around. You go ahead."

They insisted.

A golfer's mind can come up with all kinds of weird rationalizations in the course of a round. If you are playing well, the transformation in your brain goes something like this: You actually believe you are a good golfer. You believe you have the game all figured out.

And so, playing on my newfound Rocky Mountain Golf High, I teed the ball up on the fifteenth hole to show these guys some more of my golf wizardry. Because, you know, as they said, I was probably too good for them.

I never saw where my first tee shot came down; it simply disappeared high into the pine trees to the right of the fairway. I did see where my second tee shot came down; it was in the pond about 170 yards away — *on an adjacent hole far to my left.*

At times like these, I did what all elite golfers do.

"I'm just going to get out of your way, guys," I said as I scooted down the fairway without hitting another shot.

I hastily dropped a ball in the middle of the fairway and skulled that shot; it barely got off the ground. Then I did the same thing on the next shot. After a couple of chips toward the green — one too short, one too far — I grabbed my ball and dashed off the green as the two guys behind me watched from the fairway.

On the next hole, the sixteenth, I tried clearing my head, thinking the previous hole was just a crazy, bad accident brought on by the pressure of playing through strangers. But alas — *poof!* — the good golf spell had been broken. Just like that, I couldn't do anything right. I lost another two shots off the tee, dribbled my approach, and three-putted — all with those two guys watching behind me.

With my confidence shot and my equilibrium gone astray, the seventeenth hole was more of the same, and it was getting more embarrassing because my audience was two guys who once thought I was good.

But on the eighteenth hole, a majestic, straightaway par 4 that played back toward an enormous stone clubhouse, I finally hit a good drive down the middle. That tee shot left me about 160 yards to a big green, which was below a broad slate patio in front of the sprawling clubhouse.

When I got to my ball, I could see that there were people on the patio, standing and sitting around large glass tables positioned beneath outsize, festively colored umbrellas. I could hear music playing and the babble of conversation and laughter. It was a Friday evening. A cocktail party to welcome another beautiful summer weekend was in full swing.

There was a pond in front of the green, and given the way I had been playing for the last hour, I was worried about it. I turned to see that those two guys were now on the elevated eighteenth tee, looking down, waiting to see what I did. My head was swimming. The swing I thought I had been using earlier in the day had produced nothing but appalling shots for three straight holes. Just now, hitting off the eighteenth tee, I had thought nothing at all. It was entirely hit and hope.

But now what? Think about my shoulder turn? My hip drive? Keep the hands back? Keep the clubface open? Or closed? Or, maybe, close my eyes?

Times like these are the darkest, loneliest feeling in sport. You are a clueless basket case and you know it. But you have to hit another shot. People are waiting. Even though you almost can't feel your shoes walk across the grass, you must pick a club and swing.

I took a 6-iron, maybe a little too much club for the distance but I wanted nothing to do with the pond in front. "Try to stay smooth and try to relax," I said under my breath. What could go wrong? It's just a game of golf.

When I swung, I knew instantly that I hit it a little thin. This was more of a line drive than the soft, high-flying shot I envisioned. In the air, the ball was straight but kept going and going, almost seeming to gain speed as it soared over the green.

"Fore!" I yelped, knowing it was both a late warning and a futile one.

The ball struck the rigid slate of the patio on the fly, first bounding across one glass table, then ricocheting off an umbrella. It bounced all the way to the stone clubhouse wall, from which it rebounded back onto the patio where it crashed into a waitress stand and started rattling around from table to table for five or six seconds.

Standing in the fairway, I heard the sound of breaking glass. I saw startled people stumble and lurch, knocking over tables that toppled umbrellas. A waitress dropped her tray of drinks. One woman fell over backward in her chair. There was a shriek.

Then it became very quiet as every eye on the patio turned back toward the fairway where a lone figure stood holding a 6-iron.

I raced to the scene behind the green where waiters were picking up a well-dressed gray-haired woman from the patio and putting her back in her seat.

"Are you all right, Mrs. Patterson?" they said. "Can I get you anything, Mrs. Patterson? Do you want us to find your husband, Mrs. Patterson?"

I was apologizing to everyone with every step — men, women, waiters, waitresses. No one, somehow, appeared hurt or in any real distress, including Mrs. Patterson, who was busy dabbing at what looked like a cocktail sauce stain on her white skirt.

Waiters were speedily cleaning up the broken glass from the spilled waitress tray. Drinks were being refilled. Umbrellas and tables were righted, with nothing broken.

I kept scurrying around the area to see if I could help, saying, "I'm sorry" as I went and wondering if there was anything I could do. The club members, eager to get on with their weekend, were giving me a look that said, "Why don't you go away now."

Then two guys in golf attire approached me: "So, what did you hit there?"

"Six-iron."

"Way too much club," one of them answered.

"Definitely," the other said. "Are you crazy?"

I retreated from the scene, grabbed my clubs, and left them at the bag drop out by the clubhouse front door. Since my wife wasn't due for forty-five minutes, I went into the empty bar on the other side of the building. The bartender had just given me a beer when suddenly one of the kitchen staff burst in.

"Did you hear what happened on the patio?" he said to the bartender, who could not see the patio from his station.

"Some idiot flew the eighteenth green and his ball almost destroyed the whole member-guest party on the patio," the kitchen worker said. "I missed it but I heard it was amazing. Mrs. Patterson fell out of her chair."

"The club president's wife?"

"Yeah, a plate of shrimp cocktail went flying all over her."

"No kidding. She must have killed the guy," the bartender said.

"She probably would have; I think she was too startled," the kitchen worker said, then went back inside.

For the next five minutes, one by one, more kitchen help came into the bar to gossip about the near carnage on the patio.

"Somebody told me Mrs. Patterson's skirt flew over her head," one said.

"I heard she had a shrimp stuck behind her ear," said another.

I stared into my beer and moved to the end of the bar. I glanced at my watch: thirty minutes until my wife would arrive.

The hubbub seemed to be settling down when in walked the two guys who had been playing behind me.

"Hey," one said, "that was some shot you hit over the eighteenth green. Even from the tee we could see the ball bouncing everywhere. It looked like you knocked half the tables over."

"And some people, too," the other guy added.

The bartender rushed over to me, his eyes widening.

"That was you?" he asked, and when I meekly nodded, he ran for the kitchen.

For the next ten minutes, the entire kitchen workforce — along with a couple of pro shop employees — were ushered forward by the bartender, who pointed at me in astonishment.

"This is the guy who almost killed Mrs. Patterson!"

Some smiled, some shook their heads as if I was to be pitied, and some shook my hand. Every one of them asked, "What did you hit there?"

"Six-iron."

"What, are you crazy?" they said.

Finally the guys behind me turned and had another question: "You know, you were playing so well. What happened?"

I finished my beer and stood up. Heading for the door, I said: "Golf happened. I couldn't do anything wrong, then I couldn't do anything right. What happened? I was playing golf, that's what happened."

I went outside near the front portico and waited the final five minutes for my wife. When she pulled up in the car, she jumped out to help me put my clubs in the trunk.

"Hey, want to go in for a drink?" she said. "I heard they have a lovely patio in back overlooking the eighteenth hole."

Has this ever happened to you? Not the almost-killing-the-club-president's-wife part, but the part where you have a sudden, complete, and total loss of golf ability. Of course it has. The dark side of golf descends on everyone from time to time, in multiple forms. It is the golfer's nightmare: Things can and will go seriously wrong without warning.

What to do?

First, golfers should try to accept the perils of golf as a badge of honor. It is another admission ticket to the golfing tribe. You enter, have your ticket punched — feeling punched in the stomach at the same time — and you are welcomed in bittersweet melancholy. So don't fight it. Bad, annoying golf may be worrisome and unsettling, like a bad cold, but it must be endured, much like a bad cold.

Keeping with that analogy, bad golf infects almost everyone. In the very first chapter I presented some definitions of pretend golfers. Well, here's another definition of the species: Pretend golfers believe when things are going well that they have golf figured out and that things will never again spiral out of control.

Real golfers know that you never own a good, competent golf game; you only lease it. You can have a long and happy stay in the world of good golf, you might even think you have achieved a certain owner-ship status, but eventually, the lease will expire. You will be aimlessly wandering, in a golf abyss, abandoned by your clubs, your swing, your confidence, and your friends.

Sounds like fun, huh?

Cheer up.

Be reassured that since the 1500s golfers have been bothered by a sudden incapacity to do anything right. Shots that once sailed true and straight unexpectedly trail off in odd directions to distant heretofore unseen places. A sliced shot follows a hooked shot. You top a shot, instantly recall a tip about staying more on your toes to prevent thin contact, then, on your next shot, gouge a horribly fat divot that sends the ball a total of 20 yards. You hit an approach shot that misses the green but luckily stops just short of a bunker. Then you plop the next shot in the sand anyway. And take two to get out of that trap.

On the green, one putt goes halfway to the hole. The next one rockets 20 feet past the hole.

Doctors have a technical, scientific diagnosis for your condition: You have gone temporarily golf insane.

"It's not serious medically, but it's actually a fairly debilitating con-dition — at least to your golf game," said Dr. Gregg Steinberg, a sports psychologist who wrote the book *MentalRules for Golf.* "It is real; it is not imagined. At the same time, people survive it all the time, and they can return to their normal golf game faster than they think."

So it can be cured. You may have to weather a few bad times (con-sider them golf's sniffles), but you will play better again. And, by the way, don't expect too much sympathy from your playing partners. Whatever you do, don't complain to them. They will feel bad for you, again, as they would if you had a bad cold, but they also expect you to take an echinacea pill and suck it up. They know it will go away.

And that is where your recovery begins, with accepting and being buoyed by the understanding that it happens to everyone, even the best golfers in the world.

Gary Player has won nine major championships. Do you know what Player, when he was still in his prime, said about golf?

"Golf is the puzzle without an answer," he said. "I've played the game for forty years and I still haven't the slightest idea how to play."

Now, tell me, doesn't that make you feel better?

So as we tread into the dark side of golf, hoping to cast some light on its many mysteries, relax in the knowledge that every person who has waggled a club more than a hundred times has visited golf's dungeon — and lived to tell about it. And know, too, that the dark side of what can happen is both physical and mental.

But we are golfers and we are strong. We can handle anything.

Except the shanks. That leaves us weeping and useless.

The Shanks

Nothing is insurmountable, including the shanks. But it is a malady so vexing it deserves its own category of misery. At face value, a shank is a shot off the hosel, the point where club shaft meets club head. It's a pretty easy thing to do with a golf club because the center of the club-face — the optimal point of contact with the ball — may be only one-half to three-quarters of an inch from the hosel. So you're not missing by much. But when you hit the hosel and the ball goes squirting to the right (for right-handed golfers), it looks awful and it feels even worse.

A shank may be the full swing's most common malady and as such has developed its own aura of doom. A shank is so feared, golfers generally won't speak the word. Many will not even refer to it as the "*S*-word." It is so insidious golfers think it may be contagious. If you have the shanks, do not expect a friendly hug. And if you don't cure them by the end of the round, don't expect an invitation to next weekend's outing either.

But like all golf setbacks, the shanks can be overcome. The expert eye of a pro can fix it pretty quickly in most cases. And here is what some top teaching pros say they usually see:

Jim McLean is one of the biggest names in golf instruction. Incidentally, when I asked him about the shanks, he responded by giving his advice on how to cure "the heel shot." He need not speak the unspeakable. Said McLean:

"It's really a function of an outside-to-in swing path so common in many amateur players. It's like an over-the-top move only different. It often begins with a takeaway to the outside, which leads the body to feel the need to compensate. The hands and arms know things are off-line so they try to hurry the hands to the inside on the downswing. This is an effort to try to direct the center of the club to the ball. But like many compensations, it doesn't always accomplish what it hopes to accomplish. There are other things going on in the 1.5 seconds it takes to swing the golf club, and a poor takeaway eventually leads to a mishit on the heel.

"To fix this, I have my students work on a more inside takeaway path. Once they realize that coming from the outside to the inside is the problem, it solves a lot. The funny thing is they usually think they need to do the opposite to cure the heel shot."

In other words, typical of golf, people who are hitting shanks try to correct it with methods that may seem logical but, this being golf, only exacerbate the problem. For example, since you are hitting the ball off the hosel or the heel of the club, it feels as if you must be too far from the ball as you swing. So people step closer to the ball before they swing. Guess what? For many recreational golfers, that will only increase the likelihood of an outside takeaway, or an over-the-top move on the downswing, and more shanked shots.

Dave Pelz is predominantly a short-game guru, but he is also a former engineer, so when it comes to curing a golf ailment he tends to reach for personally designed props he conjured up in a lab of sorts. Here is his anti-shank suggestion:

"Find a cardboard box that is at least 6 inches high, and if you can't find a box, a bedroom pillow would work. On the practice range, place the box or pillow in line with your shoulders and feet on the ground about an inch beyond the ball. At address, the box or pillow would be almost resting on the toe of your club.

"Now make swings without contacting the box or pillow or whatever barrier you've set up — just make sure it's high enough and wide enough."

Pelz calls this homespun device "the Shanker's Delight." He recommends starting with small, shorter swings and increasing to full swings as you get good at contacting the ball rather than the box or pillow.

This is a great backyard drill done with a good practice ball or the BirdieBall.

Jim Suttie is a former PGA Teacher of the Year who instructs out of the famed Cog Hill Golf and Country Club near Chicago. Suttie says most shankers have backswings that are too flat, which means they take the club back around their body, with the club rotating more across the shoulder blades — or even closer to the waistline. At the top of the backswing, the club is often pointing well left of the target. If the target is straightaway center field, in an exceedingly flat swing, the club in the backswing is pointing toward left field. This usually leads to an open clubface going back, and an increasingly closed one on the way down.

All that club manipulation leads to several problems, and according to Suttie, a shank will likely be one of them.

So seeking help from a PGA professional might be a good idea in an overall sense. But in the meantime, Suttie has a few quick suggestions. They are easy things you can check if a spate of the shanks breaks out.

1. Lighten up your grip and hold the grip more in the fingers and not the palms of your hands. And make sure the palms face one another. This ensures that the wrists cock up and down and hinge back and forth correctly.
2. In your stance, make sure you are bent forward from the hips as well as your knees. At the same time, make sure tzhere is some room between your thighs and the handle of the club — again, to promote a more upright and less flat backswing.

3. Try to bring the club from an inside-out path on the way down to the ball. This must be really important. It seems to be part of every tip to play better golf, whether it's putting, chipping, pitching, or full shot. I guess we should work on this.

Finally, my friend Bryan Jones, with whom I have made more than fifty hysterical (if I may say so) golf videos, is the director of instruction at the David Glenz Golf Academy in northern New Jersey. During one of our videos, which depicted me developing the shanks (what great acting!) and had people running away from me like I had the plague (as if people don't do that anyway), Bryan broke down my problem. And it's a lesson he gives to many of his students.

What Bryan explained is a shanks diagnosis that focuses on the sway in a golfer's swing. We sway in lots of ways, most famously from front foot to back foot to start our swings, and perhaps worse, with our hips moving toward the target on the downswing. But what is less well known is how often many golfers sway from their heels to their toes during the swing. Said Bryan after I had shanked ball after ball:

"You have been setting up to the ball with your weight on your heels, kind of sitting back and out of balance. A lot of people do this. Maybe because one old stance tip was to pretend you're sitting on a barstool with your feet on the floor. Well, that often leads people to be too much on their heels. In that stance, you place the center of the club directly behind the ball, which is appropriate.

"The problem comes along as you begin the swing, because then you get more athletic and shift weight onto the balls of your feet, like you would in any athletic movement. But moving your center of balance moves the center of the clubface out and away from you. So instead of the club coming down to the ball at the center of the clubface, it comes down toward the heel of the club. That's a shank."

Bryan's shank antidote: "Make sure you're balanced over the center of both feet. Rock back and forth from heels to toes a few times so you can feel where the center is. You want your weight right over the arches in your feet. Now you are poised to make a balanced swing that does not sway from heels to toes, or vice versa. That makes a shank much less likely. It works, and if the shanks come back another time, you have something to try as a cure. Having something reliable to try is half the battle."

Choking

If there is another unspeakable word in golf, it is *choking.* Until Johnny Miller earned a prominent place in network golf broadcasts in the mid-1990s, you never heard the word on television when a late-round collapse was described. That is because Miller himself choked away several tournaments. He was willing to admit to it. Before Miller, the word was never uttered on television.

This was done out of a strange, golf-specific sense of courtesy. Since all golfers have choked at one time, broadcasters — who play golf — apparently felt hypocritical calling another golfer a choker.

Ken Ventura, the venerable CBS broadcaster, would never say the word no matter what happened in front of him. Scott Hoch, whose last name even rhymes with *choke,* could have won the 1989 Masters if he made a 2-foot putt. He missed it. The ball barely touched the hole at all.

I feel bad for Hoch, who lost the tournament on the next hole. I'm sure everyone feels bad for Hoch. But it was a choke. No one on the CBS broadcast ever used the word.

For decades, TV commentators — from Pat Summerall to Dick Enberg — would go to extraordinary lengths to make excuses for the world's best players, who were nonetheless choking like any other run-of-the-mill golfer. Not using the word doesn't make it go away. The game is simply too hard. People choke. Some part of the gentlemen's agreement enveloping golf — and it has value — is that sometimes you don't state the obvious. We all know a bad shot when we see it. We all know when that shot was caused by nerves and the stress of the moment.

But let's face it, when things all around you on the golf course are out of control and you're playing very poorly, a major part of the problem is mental. Can any mental issue, like choking, be overcome without stridently admitting it exists?

Sian Beilock, an associate professor in the Department of Psychology at the University of Chicago and a leading expert on human performance, apparently thinks not. She called her 2010 book *Choke*.

"I knew what I was writing about," Beilock said with refreshing candor. "I didn't see any point hiding it."

Beilock wrote more than 260 pages on the phenomenon of choking, which is something she has been studying since she first set up her own human performance laboratory. One of her favorite ways to examine what causes and can be done about choking is to study expert and beginner golfers as they putt in her lab. With the use of fMRI tests — functional magnetic resonance imaging — she can see inside the brain when golfers are trying to make short putts they would normally make with ease. She can examine how they miss and, increasingly, why they miss.

It's easy to say that we miss because the tension of the moment overwhelms us. But Beilock, who has degrees in cognitive science, kinesiology, and psychology, has been able to locate what areas of the brain are working the hardest under various specific, stressful circumstances — like making a putt under pressure. More important, she can identify what parts of the brain are getting in the way of making a simple putt under pressure. She has, in essence, identified the mental anatomy of a choke.

"The first thing to understand is that choking is a real thing, and the second thing to understand is that choking is not random," she told me. And while someone about to gag over a short putt may feel physiological effects, like sweating palms, dizziness, or trembling knees and hands, those are reactions brought about by the brain's reaction to the situation.

"You hear people who choke say afterward that they let their brain get in the way," Beilock said. "And there's truth to that. It's a little more complex but it's something like that."

Among Beilock's findings:

- Experience with performing under pressure makes a difference. Choking is not a lifetime curse. Your brain learns to react more calmly.

- Practicing under even mild pressure helps prepare you for the more intense version of a match-winning putt.
- Routine practice that has nothing to do with pressure will also hard-wire your brain to handle pressure situations.
- When faced with a pressure shot, distracting yourself from the task at hand is helpful.
- Performing quickly in pressure situations leads to more success.

"The pressure in a pressure situation is not what distracts us and makes us perform poorly," Beilock said. "The pressure makes us worry and want to control our actions too much. And you cannot think your way through a routine, practiced action, like making a 3-foot putt.

"Compare it to quickly descending a flight of stairs. You could do that without thought. But if I asked you to do it, and at the same time think about how much you bend your knee each time and also focus on what part of your foot is touching each stair, you would probably fall on your face. That's what happens when people choke. They try to think their way through the action."

As she details in *Choke*, one of Beilock's early studies of golfers under pressure involved a number of LPGA players who, while hooked up to fMRI technology, were asked to hit routine shots. Then they were asked to hit to a pin that was 100 yards away. The fMRI technology immediately detected that players with only a few years of experience activated a diffuse set of brain areas, including areas involved in fear and anxiety.

The brains of the more experienced LPGA players were considerably calmer. In a previous chapter, we talked about quiet eyes. How many athletes over the years have you heard describe a successful last-second shot by saying that in the moment they had a "quiet mind"?

It is a real phenomenon, but Beilock does not believe it is an innate skill. She instead believes the quiet-mind sensation can be learned, or at least acquired.

"There are techniques," she said. "For example, golfers have to find ways to practice pressure shots, like putts, under some pressure. Because even slight or mild pressure helps get them ready for the real thing — real pressure."

Beilock, for instance, did research in her laboratory where golfers practiced putting in front of an audience. That's mild pressure. There was no money on the putts, no punishment or penalty for missing. Humans just naturally want to do better with other people watching, and Beilock saw on the fMRI readouts that the golfers were feeling the scrutiny. More interesting, however, was that the players who putted in front of an audience were less anxious and more successful when they were asked to putt under the added stress of competition.

The putters who practiced alone did worse once they had an audience in competition.

"It happens very subtly, but understanding how your body is going to feel under pressure and learning to handle it is a skill in itself," Beilock said. "So putting yourself under even a little bit of stress when you practice can matter a lot."

Beilock suggested that golfers play games for small change with their friends on the practice putting green. If practicing alone, she said they ought to put some sort of incentive on the task, like promising to make ten 3-footers in a row before going home.

"Anything that holds you to the consequences of not succeeding will work," Beilock said.

There is proof from other walks of life that this kind of conditioning works. Soldiers training for combat are made to react over and over in tense, demanding situations. Riding in an elevator over and over makes heights less frightening to those with acrophobia.

What's most interesting is that this kind of practice actually alters the hard-wiring of the brain. It changes the neuro signals and makes the desired outcome more likely. That may sound elementary; how often have we heard the saying "Practice makes perfect"?

Beilock would rewrite that canon. Practicing under pressure acclimates you to pressure. It also builds working memory of success under pressure.

Along those lines, it's relevant to recall a conversation I had with Dr.

Charles Czeisler, who is the director of the Division of Sleep Medicine at Harvard Medical School and the chief of the Sleep Medicine Department at Brigham and Women's Hospital in Boston. Dr. Czeisler has studied a lot of professional athletes and their performance at work.

Czeisler told me how if you practice a new chipping technique for an hour but fail to get at least four hours of sleep that night, you likely won't chip any better the next day.

"That new behavior is not learned until you go to sleep," Czeisler said. "We have studied people on this and noticed that the part of the brain responsible for that new acquired skill is in a very deep sleep. It is learning the skill. People who practice it and get a good night's sleep wake up the next day and without any additional practice are 20 percent better at that skill.

"If they don't sleep, they aren't any better."

People talk about practice improving muscle memory. Practice actually improves brain memory. And you will do best if you let your brain do what it has learned and not let anything else get in the way.

There are methods for accomplishing this. In her performance lab, Beilock had golfers count backward by threes or sing a song while trying to make pressure putts. They putted better, she wrote, because they did not overthink the task at hand.

Finally, in her experiments with golfers putting in her lab, most skilled golfers putted better when instructed to putt as quickly as possible. Not hurried, just not too deliberately.

"Stepping up and putting as quickly as was reasonable was successful," she said. "We told folks to err on the side of being quick and it worked."

If you go back to the videotape of the 1989 Masters, Scott Hoch circled around his 2-foot putt twice, examining it from every angle. He took one minute and sixteen seconds to stroke the putt, which is a very long time. Too long, one suspects.

So, in the end, Beilock had several final suggestions in *Choke* for how to perform best in high-pressure athletic situations, like golf at any level of competition, including the Sunday match with your friends:

- Finding something to focus on, like the manufacturer's name or logo on the ball, might help to distract you in a productive way.
- Focus on the goal or the target, not the mechanics of what you're trying to do. Look at the back of the cup or the green; it will help you execute the practiced, acquired motor skills you have ingrained.
- Sometimes a one-, two-, or three-word mantra helps, like saying the word *smooth* while putting, or a three-word timing device during your swing, something like "back-and-through."

"People should understand that they can be more comfortable performing in stressful environments," Beilock said. "It is no different than learning to parallel-park a car. There is pressure there too, especially if it's a busy street or your spouse is in the car. But almost anyone can learn to do it."

Dr. Joe Parent is a PGA Tour instructor who has also studied choking. He has been a mental coach in golf for more than thirty years, tutoring adults, juniors, college teams, and top pros like Vijay Singh, David Toms, Juli Inkster, and Cristie Kerr.

Parent's advice on managing the mental part of your game begins with the warm-up to your round. He says golfers should begin the day putting to nowhere. By that Parent means putting to a sector of the practice green but not a hole.

"Since there's no hole, you'll make your natural stroke without pushing or pulling the putt toward the hole," he said. "You should keep doing this until you feel like you're hitting it on the sweet spot and your putts are rolling end over end. Concentrate on that feeling, not where you are hitting it."

Parent said to practice putts of varying lengths, especially some very long putts, to get a sense of pace and a feel for how big a swing of the putter you need to make to make the ball travel, say, 45 feet. That's a tough thing to do accurately on the first green without practice beforehand that day. Also, hit some putts off a side slope to get a sense for how putts are breaking and how hard you have to hit them to control and understand the break. This is good advice. How often do golfers practice breaking putts before a round?

OK, so that's a lot of putting advice, but what does it have to do with the mental game?

"It gives you confidence," Parent said. "You will have something to fall back on when you get that first breaking putt. And confidence in golf overall is very dependent on how you putt. Bad putting is very demoralizing."

Finally, Dr. Joe says to finish your putting warm-up with a series of 2-foot putts. He said while making the 2-footers to focus on keeping your head steady and listening for the putt to land in the hole. Why?

The stroke for a 2-footer is almost identical to the one you'll use for putts of 4 or 5 feet. Why listen for the ball in the hole? Because it is the sound of success. That's auditory reassurance.

Dr. Joe also counsels golfers to use self-assurance techniques when approaching every shot on the golf course. On his insightful Web site, www.zengolf.com, he quotes the great putter Bobby Locke: "Approaching a putt with doubt in your mind is nearly always fatal."

As Parent told me: "Commit to every shot. If you are wrong, you're wrong. If you don't commit, you will surely be wrong."

And finally, I think some of Dr. Joe's best advice has to do with how we carry ourselves on the golf course and how acutely it affects our play.

Parent likes to pose a question: If you stood behind the eighteenth green and watched a group of recreational golfers walking toward the green from the fairway, could you tell who is playing well and who is playing poorly? Would their posture, the pace of their gait, or something in their carriage tip off their score for the day?

Now, I know this assumes two things: recreational players walking instead of riding in a cart, and a recreational group that includes at least one golfer with a good score.

But you get Dr. Joe's point. I'm guessing that in most cases, you could tell who had a tough day — shoulders hunched, head down, walking slowly — compared to someone who was having a good, fun day — walking tall, looking straight forward, with almost a hop in the step. Your mood affects your body in very definitive ways.

It's Dr. Joe's contention that we have to avoid negative thoughts because they become a physical impediment to a good golf shot. And, it works both ways. If you are dragging yourself around the golf course, the brain and your attitude are being dragged down, too.

Instead, Parent says you should refrain from hanging your head and pull your shoulders back. Take active, deep breaths. He even suggests humming or whistling. He said to stare toward the sky, at the tops of trees, or at the horizon because it creates a constructive feeling of spaciousness.

"It helps establish a sense of the larger perspective of things," he said. "It makes it easier to go past a little setback, and it restores overall equilibrium."

Parent has also written and lectured about a small golf innovation of his: the post-shot routine. Lots of people have pre-shot routines. Do you have a post-shot routine?

"A good post-shot routine focuses on reinforcing what went well, having a sense of humor, and minimizing emotional distress about an outcome," he said. "Stay calm and look ahead to the next shot. Most of all, don't beat yourself up.

"If it was a bad shot, then the lost stroke and perhaps the bad position you now have to recover from are more than punishment enough. Don't add to it. It is going to get better."

So while we must accept that there is a dark side to this game, er, sport, we need not let it darken our door for long. When you were a kid riding the merry-go-round, did it bother you that grasping for the brass ring was so hard? No; if you missed, you waited for the carousel to spin around again for your next turn.

Golf is not unlike a ride on the merry-go-round. For four hours. I know I often leave the golf course feeling disoriented, dizzy, and maybe even a little sick to my stomach.

Just kidding. Sort of.

Perhaps Don Vickery, a teaching pro from Savannah, Georgia, said it best:

"Strange things are going to happen out there on the golf course, but golf is a game of recovery. It's not going to be perfect out there. But perfection has nothing to do with it. It's having the sense of recovery and waiting for your opportunities when they come along again."

At the time, Vickery had just become the first double amputee to earn certification as a PGA of America teaching instructor, an achievement that capped a twenty-year journey after an accident that nearly killed him.

Vickery, a fifty-one-year-old assistant professional at the Wilmington Island Club, had to pass three levels of exacting study and examination required by the PGA. Those tests included two days of golf during which he had to post a thirty-six-hole score no higher than 155. Vickery, who had one leg amputated above the knee and the other below the knee in 1989, is also missing two fingers on his left hand. With the use of leg prosthetics and a practiced grip, he shot 75 and 78.

When he got his PGA certification, Vickery said he had an overwhelming sense of gratification and accomplishment. "But mostly," he said, "I realized that golf gave me more in the last twenty years than I could ever give it."

Vickery does not easily discuss the details of his accident. "It's embarrassing," he said. "And completely my fault."

Working in construction while attending a local college, Vickery took his hunting dog for a walk on the grounds of the Fort Gordon army base near his home in Augusta, Georgia. Vickery let the dog run. "I didn't know it, but we got into a restricted area," he said. "Either he stepped on something or I did, but there was an explosion that blew my left leg off. I got hit in the chest, face, and hand, too. The dog was torn apart but still alive, and I thought at the time that my right leg was OK.

"I was bleeding pretty badly, but I tried hopping out of there carrying the dog when my right leg, which was broken, split and collapsed under me. So I was sitting there with the dog dying, and you know, you wonder just what is going to happen at that point."

A passerby saw him and summoned help.

"In the hospital, I asked the doctor if I was going to be all right," Vickery said. "And he told me: 'I don't know. You've lost a lot of blood.' I woke up a couple of weeks later, happy to be alive."

Vickery had never played golf. Growing up in a Savannah orphanage, he was a good athlete but viewed the game as "something rich people did."

He added, "Besides, it looked so easy."

The man who made his prosthetics, Ray Rice, happened to be an avid golfer. Rice suggested Vickery take up the sport.

"I said, 'Ray, I'm having a hard time just learning to walk again,'" Vickery recalled. "But I wasn't doing anything else. So I tried it. I was worried about looking silly at first, but I went out and watched able-bodied people play golf, and they looked pretty silly to me. They were hitting it all over the place."

He played every day, regardless of his pain.

"Pretty soon, I started looking forward to when I was going to play again," he said. "I came to realize pretty early that my best bet was having a strong short game, so I worked on my putting and chipping constantly. Then I went to driving ranges and watched the better players hit balls. I started trying to copy them."

Within a year, Vickery was shooting in the low 90s and landed a job at a driving range, where he mowed the grass and picked up balls.

In 1995, he returned to Savannah and went to work in the pro shop at Wilmington Island. Four years later, he was married and guiding the club's junior instruction programs when his new boss, the head pro Patrick Richardson, suggested he enter the PGA of America program and be credentialed as a golf professional.

Because the PGA certification process requires applicants to master every element of golf — swing analysis, club repair, rules, and customer service are just some of the subjects — several years of study followed. "He had a lot of support from our membership," Richardson said. "Don's an uplifting guy. I don't think I've ever heard him complain about anything. People would want to take lessons from him. Given all he's gone through, he makes a chronic slice seem like an easy thing to overcome."

Vickery now regularly visits hospitalized war veterans who have lost arms and legs.

"I go in there with shorts on, so they know that I had been in that bed twenty years ago," Vickery said. "And I say: 'Life is not over. It's going to be difficult, but not impossible. You can do anything you want. It might take a little longer but you can do it. Look at me, I'm in the mainstream of society. There's a world of people out there who will help you. You will have a life, and life will be good to you.'"

Vickery nonetheless wonders how his life might have been different without golf and all of its challenges.

"The hardest part when you lose a limb is the idleness that sets in," he said. "Golf gave me a new passion. Everything in my life at that point, even simple things, had become hard. And here was this very difficult game of golf, but there was an honor to it. I came to love the difficulty. I saw that the difficulty could be overcome.

"We are lucky to have golf. We are lucky to play it. Golf became my model for life. It's hard but I can handle it. We all can handle it. It's the mindset that changes everything. It's like I tell my students: 'Don't focus on what you can't do on the golf course. Go out there and choose to magnify the things you can do.'

"Golf is not about the mistakes you make. Golf is about the resolve you show. Those should be your proudest moments."

The Yips

There is another word that terrorizes golfers near and far, and while it is spoken from time to time, it is usually said with a raw wince or a look of shame or anguish. It is the yips, a condition where golfers flinch over short putts because their hands twitch or spasm in the putting stroke. It can be a real, definable neuro-motor hiccup in your system. It is occasionally muscular, like an overuse injury. And in some people, it is simple nervousness — trembling hands — gone to extremes. In every case, it leads to a repeated, humbling series of misses of short putts.

It is exceedingly common and has afflicted many a recreational golfer and top Tour pro alike, including major champions like Tom Watson, Bernard Langer, Ben Hogan, Lee Trevino, Johnny Miller, and Sam Snead.

Advice on curing the yips comes in many forms, and all of it might work. You need to find what seems best suited to you. All of the aforementioned golfers eventually overcame the yips.

First, I thought I would impart a little yips humor. This may be the only yips humor known to golf.

The men's pro golf tour in the 1960s was not the highly orchestrated big-money machine it is now. It was a vagabond existence, and many of the players treated it as an adventure to be savored until they went back to their less exciting lives as club teaching pros.

Guys played hard, on and off the golf course.

"It seemed like so many guys told me they had the yips back then," Jack Nicklaus once said. "Some guys really had the yips. Others just had the hangover shakes. The good putters didn't drink wine all night."

So there is yip tip number one: Don't drink wine all night. Or if you do, make sure your lagged putts end up inches from the hole.

There is other, more explicit counsel. Michael Breed, a noted teacher who has an instruction show on the Golf Channel, tells students with the yips to change putter grips. The first thing that might be worth trying is the left-hand low grip (for a right-handed putter), which is also known as the cross-handed grip. This is when your hands are inverted from the conventional putting grip. Breed also recommends the claw grip, where the left hand grips the putter normally but the right hand pinches the top of the shaft between the thumb and forefinger and the rest of the fingers rest on the side of the putter shaft. The idea is that the right wrist can no longer twist or hinge to send putts off-line.

Breed also has students try long putters, which are braced against the sternum, or medium-length putters, where the butt of the putter is positioned against the belly. Sian Beilock says trying a new grip has some scientific merit. It reprograms brain circuits, making the task seem so different that old putting problems are less likely to haunt you.

Eric Alpenfels, the putting guru from Pinehurst, has for years suggested that people with the yips look at the hole, not the ball. He also said that people who separate their hands on the putter — moving one hand down the grip so it is not touching the other hand — have had success getting rid of the yips.

Langer, the two-time Masters champion, had the yips so badly in the mid-1980s he considered quitting golf, especially after he four-putted from 3 feet at a tournament. He started experimenting. He used a conventional putting grip for long putts but went cross-handed for shorter putts. He used a long putter. He went to the claw grip.

Over time, he sufficiently distracted his mind. He made so many putts he led the European golf tour in putting.

"I still get nervous over putts, but I have the confidence that I have a way to beat it," Langer said. "If something goes wrong, I have new techniques. I think anyone who has had the yips needs to understand that you have to make changes to divert your mind. It lets you focus on what feels like a new learned skill."

David Leadbetter, who coached Langer through some of his yip problems, said the key is to find a new putting stroke that relies primarily on the bigger muscles in the body.

"That's why a belly putter or a long putter works," Leadbetter said. "You want to avoid the smaller muscles that control the wrists and hands. With the longer putters, it's a pendulum swing controlled by the shoulders. It eliminates the other muscles."

Hank Haney, Tiger Woods's former coach, has spent years studying the yips. He has seen it in junior golfers as young as eleven. He had a female student who was a surgeon. Her hands did not flinch in surgery, but they did in golf.

Haney preaches a multifaceted approach to the problem. First, he insists his students have a short but repeatable pre-shot routine, and if they develop the yips, he wants them to develop a new pre-shot routine. It can reboot the brain.

Haney also suggests trying to hit the ball on the toe or the heel of the putter because it helps the player focus on making square contact with a much smaller hitting area.

"Focusing on the smaller area keeps their minds off the overall process that brought on the yips," Haney said.

As a practice drill, he also has students putt with their driver. He has them putt balls of varying kinds and sizes: tennis balls, Ping-Pong balls, or Wiffle balls. Again, it disrupts their learned, yip-afflicted memory.

"It's not necessarily all in your mind," Haney said. "It might be neuromuscular. Sometimes I think there isn't one cause of the yips. So the cure is elusive. But there is no question that you can do things to get around it. You can work with it and succeed again. The list of great golfers who have overcome the yips is very, very long.

"What they had was the willingness to try something else. And that is what works."

All Your Other Golf-Related Problems

Some golf problems are not easily defined by unspeakable words. Sometimes, as with my long-ago day in Colorado, everything just seems to go wrong. And you are not imagining that. That's exactly what is happening.

Ask Kevin Na, a pro golfer who was ranked sixty-fourth in the world in April 2011, when he hit his tee shot on the ninth hole of the PGA Tour's Texas Open into the woods. Na chased into the woods and brambles after his ball. About five minutes and sixteen frenzied, desperate, and comical strokes later, he emerged a folk hero.

Na, who moved to California from South Korea when he was nine, took his sixteen shots without losing his ball, hitting it in a hazard, or breaking a club over his knee. He walked off the par-4 ninth hole plucking thorns and barbs from his arms and legs as his caddie brushed leaves and dirt off his back and shoulders. As I wrote in *The New York Times* two days later, the Everyman golfer rejoiced. A real golfer never gives up.

Na got a lot of credit for counting every stroke. In fact, he thought he had scored a 15, then viewed the videotape of the episode — caught on the Golf Channel — and added a sixteenth stroke. Na's misadventure was so bad it was funny.

On television, his ducking and tromping through an almost impenetrable thicket of vines, scrub bushes, and trees looked like a Golf Channel presentation of Animal Planet. All the while, because Na had agreed to wear a wireless microphone during the round, he and his caddie narrated the ruinous set of events as they unfolded.

"You've got nothing—nothing!" the caddie, Kenny Harms, said early on, weaving through the overgrowth.

"Oh, come on!" Na shouted as his eleventh shot caromed off a tree and almost hit him.

The Golf Channel broadcasters added to the sense of comedy.

"We could be here awhile," one said as Na pursued his ball deeper into the forest. Laughter can be heard in the background at times, and fans give Na a hearty round of applause when his thirteenth shot finally—and barely—flies out of the woods.

Na's troubles began when he hit his tee shot into the woods well right of the fairway. When he found his ball, he declared it unplayable. But back on the tee, Na hit what counted as his third shot into roughly the same place. He tried chipping out from the heavy brush. That shot hit a tree and struck him in the right leg, a one-stroke penalty. Na declared another unplayable lie and asked a Rules official who had burrowed into the woods after him if he could go back to the tee. That was no longer an option. He could drop in the woods.

Na turned to his caddie and said, "Kenny, just give me a ball." He was moving with great haste now, barely stopping to pause at address. He dropped the ball and hit his next shot in about five seconds. Sound familiar? Who hasn't done that? Embarrassed and infuriated, we become our own worst enemy.

In Na's case, his ball barely moved. What ensued next was even more predictable. There was a lightning-quick series of swings, so quick that PGA Tour officials later had to examine the videotape to ascertain how many times Na hit the ball. One shot went sideways, another went backward. Na, normally right-handed, swung once left-handed and missed, then swung again left-handed and made contact, but the ball did not go far. There were a couple of other off-balance swats until finally he lifted a shot just over a tree branch. The ball settled into the rough.

From there, Na hit a shot to the back fringe of the ninth green. Two putts later, he had played the ninth hole in 12 over par.

OK, so what can average golfers learn from Na's irrational five minutes?

"There comes a point when you just snap and start whaling away like Bill Murray in *Caddyshack* or something," Jim McLean said. "But that usually can be avoided if you slow yourself down. Take a walk away from the ball and gather your thoughts.

"I guess this proves even top pros can get disoriented. It's pretty impressive, though, that he finished the round strong."

And that's the rest of the story. Na went on to make three birdies and no bogeys on the back nine. He carded an 80, a truly bad round for a PGA Tour player, but it also means he was 4 under par Thursday if the ninth hole was excluded.

But there is a last bit of amusing theater to Na's golfing calamity. Asked to assess and elaborate on his day, he sounded like any other golfer.

"It was really just one bad shot," he said. "Well, two, actually. But that's what started the whole thing. It kind of gets out of hand. That's what happens in this crazy game."

Really?

But seriously, what are we to do in those circumstances and others when it feels as if you can't execute even the most simple golf shots? Phil Mickelson told me he sees it happening to amateurs in pro-ams all the time.

"A lot of people playing in pro-am events feel the pressure to do well, and when they hit a bad shot, which is going to happen inevitably, they get embarrassed and they try to make up for it by doing too much," Mickelson said. "And that usually goes bad, which leads to worse shots, and I can see it in their eyes — they're lost. It can disappear for the day if you let it."

What does Mickelson suggest?

"I ask them what their favorite club is, and I tell them to hit that almost regardless of the distance," Mickelson said. "Just take a confident swing and then do it again with the same club. Obviously, if it's a hybrid and they're only 100 yards away, that's not going to work. But many times, they can hit that hybrid off the tee and then from the fairway on the next shot. That's better than hitting a driver into a pond off the tee and then a 3-wood from a difficult lie in the rough after a drop.

"Hit a club you believe in so you can walk down the middle of the fairway and joke with the rest of us. Hitting a comfortable club for most shots over the next thirty minutes can do a lot to restore tempo and rhythm in the swing. It can save a round that was spiraling out of control."

Mike Bender, a top ten instructor who is also the personal coach to Masters champ Zach Johnson, likes the idea of playing with just one club for a while, too. Except he thinks it almost doesn't matter what the club is.

"Golfers in general would learn a lot by playing with just a 6-iron all around the golf course," Bender said. "They would come to understand how to make shots and how to manage their way around the golf course. And when things are a little out of sorts, playing with one reasonably easy-to-hit club like a 6-iron or even a 7-iron might restore some order. And it might show them how easy it can still be to score even when you don't bomb it 270 yards."

Remember, a 7-iron all around the course worked for "Tin Cup" McAvoy in qualifying for the U.S. Open.

David Leadbetter, one of the earliest coaching headliners in golf and former tutor to Nick Faldo and Michelle Wie, preaches finding the safest play available when things are going bad.

"Golf architects are not ruthless masochists," Leadbetter said. "On almost every hole, especially on the kinds of golf courses 95 percent of the golfing public plays, there is a safe place to hit the ball and it's usually a place that can be found with a routine shot.

"So I tell people, if your confidence is down, look for the widest and closest spot in the fairway off the tee. Figure out what you need to do to hit your ball to that part of the golf hole. Then, on the next shot, use the same approach mentally. You don't have to reach the green. That might be asking a little too much right now. Hit a shot that lands safely in front of the green. Next shot, more of the same — hit the simplest chip to the flattest, widest part of the green. OK, you make bogey, but you haven't made an 8. You're back in the game.

"And as you head to the next hole, do the same thing. Ask yourself: Where is the bailout spot? Because every architect built a bailout spot into almost every hole and every green. But instead, people who are struggling think they have to make up for their recent spotty play. They go for the glory shot trying to save face.

"If you're not playing with your 'A' game, that's just asking for trouble. Look for the relief on the golf course and take it. When things have brightened a bit for you, then go ahead and go for the big golf shot again."

Randy Smith, a top Texas golf teacher and coach to Justin Leonard, said he tells golfers who are going to pieces to concentrate on simple, finite body movements. Chief among them: balance.

"I tell people to take the club in balance, stay in balance, and no matter what else happens, to complete the swing with a balanced finish," Smith said. "I tell them, 'Finish with a pose just like you see the pro golfers doing on TV.' Golfers under stress get herky-jerky. They get quick. But you can't just say, 'Slow down.' Because the golf swing is a fairly abrupt athletic movement. Saying, 'Slow down' can cause other problems."

Mike LaBauve is also one of the nation's top golf teachers, and his wife, Sandy, is another top one hundred golf instructor. I've always wondered what their dinnertime conversations are like.

"Not always golf," Sandy said. "But we might go over things that happened that day. We'll talk about what students we had, what they needed to work on. Some things are eternal — how to get them to practice their putting more, how to get people to think about where the clubface is in the swing."

Between them, the LaBauves have witnessed myriad instruction trends and counseled countless golfers trying to find their way in this maddening game. What is their advice on what to do when golf's demons seem to be winning on the golf course?

"I think some of it is accepting that bad things are going to happen and to be prepared for it," Sandy said. "Don't get upset by it. Unless you break 80 regularly, you're going to make a lot of mistakes. One way to learn to deal with them is to not let the mistakes take you by surprise. Instead, be prepared for them."

Added Mike: "If you're a 20 handicap, you should be ready to miss more than three-fourths of all greens. But you would be a 10 handicap if you knew what to do next and had repeatedly practiced those short shots near greens after a miss. Be ready for misses."

As LaBauve points out, even PGA Tour players miss about six greens in regulation per round. A 20-handicap golfer misses on average about fourteen greens in regulation per round, he estimated.

"Understanding and accepting that you are going to make mistakes is a big part of getting better," said LaBauve, who is the director of instruction at the Westin Kierland Resort and Spa in Scottsdale, Arizona. "The key is to perfect short-game shots for those mistakes and you'll see incredible improvement — from six to ten shots per round, depending on your handicap."

If all else fails, I offer this last word from Mickelson, who finished in the top ten of a major championship seventeen times before 2004 but never won one. At the Masters tournament, he had been the third-place finisher three times. In 2004, he finally won his first major, then won twice more in the next six years. On the subject of playing through a golfing funk, or perhaps speaking about overcoming hardship in general, Mickelson smiled and said, "It is always darkest before dawn."

My wife and I didn't have that drink on the infamous patio of that picturesque club in Colorado those many years ago, but I want to tell you about the round of golf I played just a few days later, at a different club. After an admittedly shaky start, I was playing well — not spectacularly, but good enough. I was by myself again and finished out the round on the eighteenth hole, when, as if by fate, I had an approach shot of about 160 yards to the green.

There was water in front of the green. There was a clubhouse behind the green. There was a courtyard with tables and umbrellas in front of the clubhouse. (What is it with these Colorado golf courses?)

Looking toward the green, in my mind's eye, I could see a golf ball bouncing all over the place. I could see umbrellas toppling. I could hear the broken glass. I could see Mrs. Patterson, except this time she was shaking a fist at me.

I knew this was one of those pivotal athletic moments. I had to persevere. I could not let golf's dark side continue to rule. I had to face the challenge and succeed.

So, what did I do?

Maybe you think I hit it pure and left it 4 feet from the hole. Sure, I hit a 6-iron.

In fact, instead I took my 7-iron and aimed left of the green where there was a little grassy collection area — a bailout spot. It was bathed in sunlight, a beacon of hope. I swung and watched the ball safely land there. Then I chipped up to 3 feet and made the par putt.

I plucked my ball from the hole, shouldered my bag, and walked toward the courtyard, where two women sat sipping cocktails.

"Thought you were going to go for it back there," one said.

I stopped.

"Are you crazy?" I said.

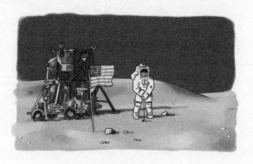

13

Nine Places Every Golfer Should Play

*The ardent golfer would play Mount Everest
if somebody put a flagstick on top.*

PETE DYE

GOLFERS ARE CREATURES of habit. Ever watch some people go through their pre-shot routine?

Tug on the glove, adjust the belt, position the left foot, then the right foot, pull on the pant leg, look at the target once, reposition the feet, look at the target again, flex the knees, bend the elbows, look at the target again . . .

OK, you get the idea. Didn't mean to make you want to scream, "Hit the ball!"

My point is that golfers like routines. There is comfort in them. It's bred into us, like an inherited territorial trait. It's why people who visit a classroom a second time most likely will gravitate toward the seat they sat in during their first visit. It's why people in office complexes, without realizing it, try to put their car in the same parking spot day after day.

And so it is with golf courses. People go back to the same ones over and over. There is nothing wrong with this. It's fun to know the twists and turns of every hole in a favorite layout. It's a challenge to find new ways to conquer those holes. And, of course, it's good for your score to know the breaks in each green.

But golfers can take the desire for familiarity too far. There are 16,000 golf courses in the United States alone, but many recreational American golfers, perhaps even a majority, play 80 or 90 percent of their rounds on two or three of the same golf courses. A routine is understandable, but the banquet of golf offerings is too great to sample from the same plate day after day.

Now, it's understandable that most golfers can't travel the world to find new, exotic golf courses to add to their personal collection. I concede that people often play at the same places because it is easy and economical.

But to embrace the lifelong golf experience, you must branch out, and I am not talking about playing as many golf courses on the *Golf Digest* top hundred list as possible. This is not a chapter about great golf courses few can play, or great golf courses that cost $300 or more to play. You can find that list anywhere. Nor is this a chapter about nine specific golf courses every golfer should play. It is not a chapter about specific golf courses at all, or at least not many of them. What I want to do is underscore the wonderful bounty and variety of golf courses available to just about everyone. I'm talking about mom-and-pop golf courses, real and faux links courses, and demonic Pete Dye layouts. There is precious, lost golf architecture and plenty of quirky gems to be found off the beaten track.

The dimensions of a baseball diamond, a football field, a soccer pitch, or a tennis, squash, or basketball court are nearly always the same. And they are basically flat as well. But golf is played under the most changeable conditions with courses that can be thousands of yards longer with different species of grass and trees. Some are hilly, some are by the sea, and some are inland. Nothing is consistent, even about the same golf course, day to day. And golfers need to celebrate those differences by seeking out the adventure of golf.

This is the chapter that embraces that versatility and encourages golfers to discover the sport's diversity, from oceans to snowfields.

Golf, if it is not obvious by now, is not to be played in the finite bubble of uniformity. That would be too easy. Golf is more like mountain climbing where the courses are ascents to be claimed and remembered. Each climb teaches you something. And when you are at the top, the view is worth savoring. Take it all in; it's a big world.

So, here are nine places every golfer should play. Why nine? Why not ten, like David Letterman's lists? Because Letterman isn't a golfer. Golfers think in nines. To wit:

1. Nine-Hole Golf Courses

The most unheralded resources of American golf are the plucky nine-holers, many of them designed before an officious, late-twentieth-century snobbery put an unwarranted emphasis on the eighteen-hole golf course. As of 2011, there were still more than 4,400 nine-hole golf courses in the United States, which make up about 28 percent of all golf facilities. And yet, there hasn't been a nine-hole golf course listed in the major golf magazines' best one hundred golf course rankings since 1968.

It's a silly oversight. And it turns our back on the history of the game, especially in this country. When golf was introduced to America in the late nineteenth century, nobody was building eighteen-hole golf courses. They were not going to devote the extra money and land it took to construct an eighteen-hole layout for what might be a sporting fad.

Golf courses are eighteen holes in length because, since 1764, that's how many holes St. Andrews in Scotland has had. If the Scots trying to organize and bring uniformity to the game back then had picked a different year or a different course, the standard golf course length might be twenty-two holes, or fourteen. Anyway, eighteen holes does usually seem to be just about the right number. But not always. And it doesn't mean you have to play eighteen entirely different holes to have a good golf round.

The first United States Open, in 1895, was played on a nine-hole golf course. They played the nine holes at the Newport Country Club in Rhode Island twice. Until the late 1920s, the majority of new golf courses were still of the nine-hole variety. Some of the greatest golf courses designed by some of the greatest architects, like Donald Ross, were nine-hole designs.

So it's important to understand that nine holes does not mean half as good. The understated nine-hole golf course at the east end of town might be twice the challenge and twice as inventive as the lavish eighteen-hole golf course at the west end of town.

What sets nine-hole courses apart is usually the historical origin and the genial attitude of the place. They are most often decidedly unpretentious. With smaller budgets and less land and without heavy machinery, the builders of nine-hole courses were often forced to keep quirks of the natural landscape in play instead of bulldozing them as many 1980s and 1990s designers did. So you see things like double greens, swamps, or massive trees smack-dab in the middle of the fairway or a routing with back-to-back par 3s. You play these courses and find yourself saying things like "I've never seen that before." And that's the point.

Many nine-hole golf courses also were built before the widespread use of carts, and that influences the way they play—they're easier to walk, and the green complexes aren't constructed to kowtow to the almighty cart path. That means greens are irregular shapes placed in irregular places. That makes the golfer hit shots that might not seem so routine. And that's a good thing. Unlike its eighteen-hole brethren, the nine-hole golf course is not trying to conform to the standard notion of what a top golf course is supposed to look like. The nine-hole golf course is the humble little barbecue hut that all the locals visit. It doesn't look like much, but it's fabulous once you get to know it. And everybody keeps coming back.

Nine-hole golf courses are a state of mind, a chance to walk away from the conventional. Wherever you live, I bet there is a great nine-hole course waiting, perhaps idly, to be discovered.

This is not to denigrate eighteen-hole golf courses. Most golf is and should be played on eighteen-hole golf courses. The genius, splendor, and tradition of the game's most esteemed full-scale layouts provide a separate joy. But golf on America's nine-hole courses is too important to ignore. It is the land as it was; it is golf as it was.

Some people will tell you that nine-hole golf courses are on their way to obsolescence, and indeed, more than 1,000 have closed or converted to eighteen-hole courses in the last several decades. The modern golf world has grown bigger and longer — be it the size of a typical driver head or how far a ball travels — and golf courses have ballooned with the trend. But this is not necessarily progress. As with many things, less can be more in a golf course.

Having grown up playing nine-hole golf courses in New England, I have always sought them out. You also never know what you're going to stumble upon at a nine-hole golf course, which is part of the charm. I have played around and over Revolutionary War–era stone walls that bisect fairways or hide greens. I have played from a tiny island tee box in a tiny pond accessed by a tiny rowboat (choose your club wisely, because you're not going back for another). I have played to greens positioned 90 feet below the fairway.

Nine-hole courses also allow golfers to discover the hidden gems of our most noted pre-Depression-era golf architects, since all of them cranked out nine-hole courses.

Several Ross designs have been preserved in New England, and Robert Trent Jones's creativity and subtlety are still evident in nine-hole designs from Illinois to New York. One of those Ross designs is in the foothills of the Catskill Mountains, in Palenville, New York, about one hundred miles northwest of New York City at the public Rip Van Winkle Country Club. Designed by Ross in 1919, it is laid out beneath a striking mountain ridgeline. Greens fees have been about $15 on weekdays and $20 on weekends for years.

If you think the nine-hole golf course is an evolutionary dinosaur, you need to visit a place like the Rip, as locals call it.

"As a business model, I much prefer having nine holes," said John Smith, the third generation in his family to run the Rip.

"Expanding to eighteen holes would be the last thing I would do," Smith, who is in his mid-thirties, said. "My taxes, my fuel costs, my employee expenses, and my maintenance budget would double. I've known a lot of nine-hole golf courses that have converted to eighteen holes. I know for certain that they are not bringing in double my revenue."

Smith, whose grandfather bought the club in 1949, concedes that potential customers call him every day to ask how many holes the Rip has. When they hear nine instead of eighteen, "sometimes they hang up without saying a word," he said. "We know there's a stigma."

But he also knows there are people who don't have the time to play eighteen holes, and people who can't physically play eighteen holes. There are also people who know that playing from his course's two sets of tees alters the driving strategy enough that eighteen holes on the same nine feels almost like any conventional course.

"Some people prefer the more laid-back atmosphere of a nine-hole golf course," Smith said. "They know they're not going to get pushed around here. Nobody is going to hurry you."

About a ninety-minute drive from Rip Van Winkle, the Hotchkiss School nine-hole golf course in Lakeville, Connecticut, was built by noted golf architect Seth Raynor in 1924. A recent *Golf World* article ranking the top twenty-five nine-hole courses in the country — yes, there is such a thing — listed the Hotchkiss course at number 22. The Hotchkiss layout has devilishly sloping fairways, spectacular lake views, and a closing-hole par 5 that begins in a narrow stand of trees, skirts past a swamp, and finishes with a serpentine uphill approach to a plateau green. There's a little clubhouse behind the green, and a bunch of regulars were waiting to start their weekly league as I finished playing there one summer day a few years ago. They sat on benches watching people like me try to survive the final hole.

When I was done, they seemed to acknowledge the surprise in my eyes, smiling as if to say, "And you thought this was just a harmless little nine-hole golf course, didn't you?"

If you don't regularly play nine-hole golf courses, that is what you are missing. And you might want to play them while there are still so many available. Some nine-holers in future years will close because they are not well run, well maintained, well located, or well designed in the first place. We won't miss those tracks.

But thousands of distinctive nine-hole courses continue to thrive, like an alternative wing in the house of golf. People go there not to be seen, not for ultrapristine conditions, not for excessive length, and certainly not to be wowed by the nineteenth-hole catalog of $8 beers.

We go there to play and, in a sense, to be around others with the same simple aspiration.

The desire and need for a golf course with a short list of goals — playable, enjoyable, congenial — will never go away. A lot of us began playing on nine-hole courses. A lot of us like to find our way back to them. They are familiar and soothing, like walking through your home's front door after a long trip.

The last time I played at Rip Van Winkle, I was with my son, Jack, who was eleven at the time. At the beginning of our round, a dog lazily chased a deer across a fairway. Two ducks quacked at the commotion at the Rip. It is quiet and busy at the same time. At one point, Jack took three swipes to get out of a bunker. He couldn't care less that this was taking extra time, and neither could the group behind us — wherever they were.

By the fifth hole, I don't think we were keeping score anymore. I don't remember. I do remember the view back up the fairway as the sun put a glow on clouds disappearing behind the mountain ridge. I remember my son making an improbable 30-foot downhill putt, and when he let out a yelp, I remember a fish jumping in a nearby pond. I remembered why I play golf.

2. Pete (and Alice) Dye Courses

If playing a nine-hole golf course is like going home, then playing a Pete and Alice Dye golf course is the direct opposite, unless you grew up in a circus fun house.

I've played golf with Pete Dye, the mad scientist of golf architecture, a few times — always on one of his devilish golf courses. I don't ever recall shooting a decent score, and yet I don't recall ever having more fun. I've played his golf courses without him as a partner, too. And as I flailed through those typical Dye humps, swales, and nasty par-3 water hazard holes, I sometimes recorded double-digit scores on a hole or two. But I still had a good time. Playing and thinking your way around a Dye course is one of golf's most fulfilling challenges. And that's what makes Pete, and his golf courses, a gift to the game. Because his courses are so prized and well regarded, many have become a little pricey to play, but every serious golfer should play as many of them as is reasonable for time, travel, and budget. Keeping to his simple roots, most Pete Dye courses are open to the public.

Playing a Dye golf course is connecting to the game and rewarding its growth in the 1970s and 1980s, because the Dyes helped usher in a new era of bold and daring golf architecture.

Railroad ties used to buttress and beautify greens near water hazards? Those are a Dye invention. Scary and expansive bunker complexes? Few were ever as daunting or eye-catching as the ones Dye designed. They were dubbed "golf eye candy." Quirky tee boxes that rise out of wetlands, giving the golfer uncommon sightlines? That's pure Pete Dye. Tall wild fescue and twisting, testing fairways that resemble Scotland but still somehow remain uniquely American? It's a Dye trademark. Grass mounds and hollows that replaced sand bunkers? That's a Dye trick. It looks easier than a ball being in the sand. (It isn't.) Devilish par-3 holes that are Dye-abolical for the variety of ways they can be played — with good results and decidedly bad ones? Every Dye course has two or three.

For these reasons and many more, you should find a Dye design near your home. Chances are you won't have to go too far. You won't be sorry.

Well, actually, at some point on some hole you will probably be very sorry, and you will surely feel cursed, but in the end you will have visions of dozens of memorable shots. And isn't that the measure of a great golf course?

Pete, who is in his mid-eighties and regularly shoots better than his age, likes to say that he enjoys entertaining guests on his golf courses. He always has breakfast or lunch with them before the golf round.

"That's because they aren't speaking to me after they play," he says.

The fact is, Pete sits down with you after the round, too. He wants to hear the feedback. He is too much of a polite midwesterner, the kind of guy who would sit in your living room and attentively sell you a life insurance policy.

Because that is, in fact, what Pete Dye did for the first ten years of his professional life. He was the best life insurance salesman in Indianapolis. Pete and his wife, Alice, have been iconic figures in the golf community for so long it's hard to recall from whence they came. And it's hard to remember how much in disarray American golf architecture had become in the mid-1950s.

"Golf architecture was not a profession at all," said Alice Dye, who married Pete in 1950. She has since won two national amateur championships and been a prominent golf administrator and author. "There was once a boom in golf course development, but it died out during and after World War II. The few men still designing golf courses told us not to bother trying. They said we would starve our two children."

But Pete was bored selling insurance. So they designed and built public golf courses for $2,000, or less. Pete gave up his $35,000 salary for an annual income of $5,000.

Pete went to college at night, taking courses in agronomy, turf management, and irrigation techniques. He and Alice joined the USGA's green section committee and took a lengthy trip to Scotland and Ireland, where they visited all the historic courses and took copious notes. And slowly, they unleashed their new vision for American golf at what became important golf crossroads: the Harbor Town Golf Links in Hilton Head, South Carolina; the Crooked Stick and the Brickyard Crossing golf courses in Indiana; the Honors Course in Tennessee; and, of course, TPC at Sawgrass in northern Florida, home of the iconic island green seventeenth hole.

In 1989, he agreed to build a golf course on Kiawah Island because the site had been awarded the 1991 Ryder Cup matches. His partners in the venture owned a piece of oceanfront property and not much else.

"Reporters at the press conference announcing Kiawah as the Ryder Cup site asked me where I was going to put the galleries," Pete said one day in 2010, sitting in his Florida living room. "And I said: 'Galleries? I don't even know where the holes are going yet.'"

Dye did lay out the holes, until Hurricane Hugo destroyed all that work. It didn't matter. Dye had Kiawah Island's Ocean Course ready for perhaps the most famous Ryder Cup ever — the War on the Shore that turned the Ryder Cup into a major international event. The Ocean

Course, with Dye's distinctive undulating fairways and peekaboo greens, is consistently rated one of the top five public golf courses in America.

But you don't have to go to exclusive Kiawah Island to find Dye masterpieces — although Kiawah is a wonderfully indulgent golf destination. The Dyes made dozens of golf courses for the people. There are Dye courses in twenty-eight states and five foreign countries. When you play them, not only do you celebrate the rebirth of American golf architecture — dormant during the wartime economies of the 1940s and early 1950s — you also celebrate a prized golf partnership. Pete Dye has built most of his courses by moving there to be with them as they mature. He and Alice brought their two sons, P. B. and Perry, along for the ride, hopscotching around the country. Not surprisingly, P. B. and Perry are now golf architects, too.

Alice was president of the American Society of Golf Course Architects for many years and influenced many a Dye design. In fact, when Pete was inducted into the World Golf Hall of Fame in 2010, he joked, "I'm still not sure you're inducting the right Dye."

"There are three things that matter most about a golf course," Alice said when I played a round with her in 2008 (she also shot better than her age). "The first thing is, Does it make you think? The next is, Does it make you smile? And the last is, Does it make you want to come back?"

Dye golf courses are usually taxing and difficult. People rarely shoot career lows. And yet, people flock to them. They are more than badges of honor. People want to be engaged by the golf course, and the Dyes will not disappoint in that interaction. There is genius, daring, and innovation at a Dye-designed course. Go there to think, smile, and ponder when you will come back.

3. Golf Courses Not Designed by Big-Name Architects (but by Some Forgotten Ones)

Kent Lemme, the superintendent at the venerable Taconic Golf Club in Williamstown, Massachusetts, gets the same question all the time: "This course is a Donald Ross design, right?"

Impressed by a classic layout, golfers routinely invoke the name of Ross, an icon of early-twentieth-century golf course architecture.

Lemme has a stock answer: "No, this course is a Stiles and Van Kleek."

"People say, 'A what and what-what?' Nobody has heard of those guys," Lemme said.

The more you play golf, the more you start to appreciate the impact quality golf architecture has on your enjoyment of a round. It's more than mounds, sand, and tilted greens; superior golf design sculpts and shapes your passage through the day. The setting becomes the experience.

In recent decades, just as baseball fans learned to treasure the timeless character of Fenway Park or Wrigley Field, there has been nostalgia for the enduring work from golf's Golden Age of architecture, roughly defined as the period from 1910 to the late 1930s. Before the Golden Age, most American golf courses were primarily functional. Holes would be plainly practical. It was obvious what the straightest approach to the hole would be; the golfer's test was to follow that most direct course. Golden Age architects introduced intricate strategies by having most holes bend around natural features in the landscape. Cleverly placed hazards created risk/reward options both off the tee and when approaching the green. Holes could suddenly be played in multiple ways. It was up to the golfer to decide how to attack each hole — and hope he or she was not being deceived into the wrong choice.

Some of the names that dominate this era are Ross, Alister MacKenzie, and A. W. Tillinghast. You will rarely hear the names of their contemporaries Wayne Stiles and John Van Kleek. The same goes for William Langford, another largely undervalued architect from the era. Many lesser-known modern architects are equally overlooked, such as Stephen Kay.

It should be said that it is the serious golfer's job to find the designs of these forgotten or underappreciated masters. It may not have the same impact on your friends as telling them you just played a Dye design or one by Robert Trent Jones Jr., and obviously those courses have a significant appeal. But finding the unseen has its own appeal, and it might be more fun because you will know you have uncovered something that is there in plain sight. It is a personal delight, and if you keeping looking, you will see that their work is almost everywhere.

Consider the Boston-based Stiles, who designed more than 140 courses from Maine to New Mexico in the 1920s and 1930s. More than 70 remain, including many memorable layouts throughout New England. Van Kleek, his partner for several years, designed courses all over the world and in the mid-1930s was the supervising architect for a renovation of the New York City Parks Department's golf offerings. Van Kleek put his stamp on golf courses throughout New York, from Split Rock in the Bronx to the Clearview layout in Queens — with Dyker Beach and Van Cortlandt Park in between.

"Stiles and Van Kleek weren't splashy, self-promoting guys," said Bob Labbance, who wrote the book *The Life and Work of Wayne Stiles*, along with Kevin Mendik. "They didn't do many big, expensive projects. They pleased their clients and their communities with relatively low-cost golf. But play those courses today and you appreciate the craft and talent involved."

More than eighty years after their creation, by meandering down a quiet road, you can find these Stiles and Van Kleek jewels waiting to be discovered. A few years ago, I created my own Stiles and Van Kleek golf trail, visiting three beautiful public golf courses separated by no more than twenty-five miles along Route 7 in the Berkshire Mountains of Massachusetts, about a two-and-a-half-hour drive north of New York City.

My first stop was the Cranwell Resort, Spa and Golf Club in Lenox, designed in 1926. Stiles, who began his career as a landscape architect, looked at the inspiring stone mansion that dominates the property and cleverly built some holes around it. But on the back nine, Stiles, who did most of the design work for the Massachusetts courses, took the golfer on a captivating trip through verdant woods.

Stiles liked to create golf holes that existed in their own setting, independent and unseen from other holes on the course. At Cranwell, hole after hole on the back nine appears around every bend, each a distinct challenge and each with a slightly different look from the previous holes. Slipping through the woods to play the Cranwell back nine is an entertaining trip through a landscaper's labyrinth.

Like most Stiles and Van Kleek courses, Cranwell is not overly long and has open and accessible fairways off the tee. As Geoff Schackelford wrote in his insightful book *The Golden Age of Golf Design,* the Golden Age architects liked to let golfers keep the ball in play off the tee. It lets more people in on the golf adventure to follow. And that is true at Cranwell, where, for example, a drive down the middle put me in good position on the fourteenth hole. But once the ball is safely in play, that's when the fun begins.

On the fourteenth, as in many Stiles and Van Kleek designs, the fairway slants in the same direction as the green, adding a double challenge to an approach shot. Stiles and Van Kleek courses are usually playable for golfers of all abilities because almost everyone can get approach shots to the greens or at least near them. But there is still a catch: Only those positioned in the right place will have any chance at par. Like at the Cranwell's fourteenth, which demands that you hit a draw off a slice lie to a green designed to repel any shot with the slightest slice.

"Stiles always found his green sites first, then worked backward from there," Mendik said. "And as a landscape architect, he knew what the trees on a hole would look like in sixty or eighty years. He saw the whole picture."

A short drive north from Cranwell to the town of Dalton is the Wahconah Country Club, which like Taconic is semiprivate. Stiles came to the site in 1928, and he and Van Kleek were paid $37,500 to lay out what is now the front nine of eighteen holes. These holes have signature Stiles and Van Kleek traits: elevated greens and back-to-front sloping greens. Wahconah is also known for being the location of the last round played by Bobby Jones, on August 15, 1948.

The Taconic Golf Club, the most decorated Stiles and Van Kleek course, is the farthest north and is owned by Williams College, one of the nation's finest liberal arts colleges. Built on farmland, it has a parklike feel, with a familiar, pleasing routing to the holes and lightning-fast, tilted greens. I had a 10-foot downhill putt on the thirteenth hole that did not look hard. My next putt was 35 feet back up the hill. On the fourteenth tee, there is a plaque commemorating a hole in one recorded by Jack Nicklaus during the 1956 United States Junior Amateur. That is the best way to avoid putting at Taconic.

While Stiles and Van Kleek were shaping intriguing golf courses in mostly northeastern states, William Langford, with partner Theodore Moreau, was creating about 200 courses in the Midwest. Two decades after his work was complete, two other midwesterners, Pete and Alice Dye, were touring the Langford sites. Langford's ideas were a big influence on the Dyes as developing golf architects.

Langford's routings were different from those of Stiles or Van Kleek because he would usually first identify the most valuable land for fairways and build greens later. Langford did this largely because of where he was designing his golf courses. In the Midwest, he had vast stretches of land and horizons that seemed to go on forever. How could he create golf holes that were not overwhelmed by their surroundings?

His answer was to mold majestic fairways that took in the big valleys and ravines. Langford holes were brawny and bold, like the landscape. He liked to curve par-5 fairways in an *s*, like a switchback curve on a European mountain road. That would make golfers have to consider hitting the ball left to right and then right to left.

A lot of people don't know the Langford name but they should. His best course is Lawsonia in Wisconsin, consistently rated one of the best in the Midwest. Other Langford designs are sprinkled throughout the region, like the Wakonda Club in Des Moines, which is a challenging, difficult layout, one that has been lengthened but still has the look and feel of a course opened in 1922.

Langford also created Harrison Hills Golf Club in Attica, Indiana, which was carved into hilly terrain that spawned severely undulating greens. Other Langford layouts are near Chicago (Skokie Country Club) and Omaha (Happy Hollow Golf Course).

It is not only those forgotten that get overlooked. In plain sight, people ignore gifted designers like Stephen Kay.

The best thing about a Kay design is that it is intentionally understated. At the opening of the Links at Union Vale, a new public course forty miles north of New York City, Kay said he considered it a compliment when a golfer has to ask who the course designer is.

"I don't want my ego stamped on the land and the course," said Kay, who has designed dozens of courses nationwide. "We strive for playability, beauty, safety, and acceptance of all levels of golfers. And we use different techniques for different landscapes."

Kay designed a little, flat nine-hole public course in my hometown. There is a tiny sign designating it as a Stephen Kay effort. But the place, thankfully, is almost always packed.

All too often, designers like Kay, Stiles, Van Kleek, and Langford are the small-print names in a world of big-name golf course architects. Don't fall into the trap of chasing only the noted designers. Golf is not like buying jeans or a camera, where the well-known big-box stores have better prices and a better selection. If anything, it can sometimes be the other way around.

Do a little homework and learn about the other gifted designers from the Golden Age and beyond. They left golfers a legacy of fun, playable courses to discover. It is up to us to remember their names in the search.

4. Good Miniature Golf Courses

It is stunning how many serious golfers never play any serious miniature golf. This is a major mistake. Golf is not meant to be played in long form only. Miniature golf is great putting practice, it broadens your golf creativity, and you might win a free ice cream cone on the last hole.

Does your country club do that for you?

Now, it's important that it be a quality miniature golf course. There are some poorly maintained ones. But there is a growing subset of clever, testing, and imaginative miniature golf courses. And that, my fellow golfer, is an altogether different golf game. In fact, there is even a professional miniature golf circuit, the U.S. Pro Mini Golf Tour.

"People laugh when I tell them I am a professional mini golf player,"

Peter Gilchrist of Boothbay, Maine, said. "I can't get upset at them. I know a lot of people don't take mini golf seriously. Although we do."

One person's leisurely respite puttering around while on vacation is another person's workday passion. The miniature golf land of pirate ships, castles, windmills, and jungle volcanoes — Americana by the roadside — is the setting for heated and earnest competition in dozens of cities and towns across the country. Men and women are ranked nationally and travel to tournaments days in advance to chart the courses, practice eight hours a day, and plot strategies for getting an ace on every hole. Some players carry their specially crafted putters in gold cases, and others keep their golf balls in boxes like humidors to regulate temperature and ensure consistent bounces off brick or stone railings.

There's a fifty-page mini golf tour rule book, which includes an antidoping clause and a dress code: collared shirts and no sandals.

"I know it sounds crazy, but you can't just walk out there and compete with the mini golf pros," said Gilchrist, who is in his sixties and owns a restaurant in Maine. "If some guy from the PGA Tour came to one of our events and tried it without practicing for at least a month, he would be humiliated."

Gilchrist and his wife, Nancy, have each won a national mini golf championship. So have their son, Peter, and their daughter, Alice.

Tom Dixon, a Missouri truck driver who arranges his cross-country deliveries around his annual thirty-five-tournament mini golf schedule, added: "People laugh at us and say, 'What's so hard about hitting it through the clown's nose?' I tell them to come out and try playing with us. We get those cocky first-timers in tournaments and usually beat them by twenty shots."

Now, I know what you're thinking: Come on, how hard can this be?

First of all, the winners of professional mini golf events often average about thirty strokes per eighteen holes throughout a taxing, six-round tournament. They play on unpredictable courses that customarily require more skill than the average roadside miniature golf course — although there are still holes where you putt the ball through the front door of a haunted house and wait for it to come out the other side.

But many modern and progressive mini golf courses now resemble real golf courses except in miniature, with water hazards, sand traps, elevation changes, and obstacles like rock outcroppings. The pros also worry about varying carpet surfaces and hidden, subterranean breaks based on faults in the cement or concrete below the hole.

"Basically, you have to map out every hole in a notebook days ahead of time," said George Tarrant, a pro mini golfer from Florida.

The professional mini golf scene is big enough to have not one, but two national tours, and they have occasionally clashed. Between the two groups, about 500 mini golf pro players pay between $40 and $75 each in annual association dues. There are several competition categories, including junior, senior, and amateur divisions. Men and women compete against one another in the open division, and dozens of players from Europe, where competitive mini golf is more popular, fly in for the American events. Prize money was once as high as $50,000. Lately, winners receive about $1,500 — still not bad pay for hitting a golf ball thirty times within 30 square yards.

There is a United States Open of mini golf and a Masters tournament, too.

So what can we learn from these gurus of the perfect putt?

"The putter itself doesn't matter that much," said Gilchrist, who has won several national titles using an $8 putter, like the kind you rent with a purple ball at the mini golf counter. "It's about a calm stroke. Low and slow and the ball will roll true."

Mini golf pros said regular golfers should go to the miniature golf course to improve their concentration on the greens.

"Not enough regular golfers realize that putting is actually a separate game of golf," said Dixon. "Ben Hogan said that because putting was so much harder for him than swinging the club. It's true for a lot of people.

"But if they went to the miniature golf course, they might start to see putting as more fun. It's not torture. Anybody can learn to do it better."

One miniature tip for the big course from Dixon (who is a 9 handicap in "big" golf): "When I play regular golf, I'm amazed at how little concentration people put into their putting. They take a couple of practice strokes with their putters, but you can see they really aren't focusing on things like the speed of the putt. They look at the hole but not the distance to the hole.

"I'm amazed at how often putts are either short of the hole or way past it. I think people rush and just hit it. In mini golf, we know that speed control is everything."

Several mini golf pros said they thought that regular golfers might be so distracted or frustrated by the time they reach the green that giving their undivided attention to putting is difficult, if not impossible.

But in mini golf, you are always putting. So you might learn something you can bring to the big course.

"There's no question, when you come to a mini golf course, where you can't lose your ball in the woods or hit a shot out-of-bounds, it's much easier to focus on the act of rolling a little ball a relatively short distance along the ground," Gilchrist said. "It centers people on the basics of the task. It may not be easy to be a great putter, but it's not hard to be a decent putter.

"Just get out on our carpets and give it a try."

5. Links-Style Courses, Even if They Are Not "True" Links (Don't Let the Links Snobs Keep You Away)

It is a truth in the golf world that there are a limited number of authentic links courses, generally defined to mean courses on land that is coastal, flat, and of no agricultural value — a strip of land that is a *link* from the sea to more fertile land. Other conditions have been added to the definition in some quarters. A true links course has dunes, undulating topography, and sandy soil. And since trees will not usually grow in those conditions, treeless is a likely feature of a true links course. And without trees, wind is likely.

OK, so we understand there are some pure, established links course settings.

Now, here comes the problem. In the United States, there is only so much coastal land that was left to golf course development. Unlike the land along the North Sea in Scotland, some of our barren seacoast is still pretty close to major American cities, so a lot of that land was used for its fantastic real estate value. But American golf course designers still wanted to create links golf courses. Or at least links-style golf courses.

And we have created them. Many are treeless and windy and have some of the flat land features and big greens where the best play is to run the ball up along the ground. They are very different from the target golf, mountain golf, desert golf, or parkland golf that most Americans expect.

Still, to purists, they are not technically a true links. I agree. So that's why people call them links-style golf courses. But don't let anyone dissuade you from playing them just because they are not the same as what's played in Scotland. If you can drive an hour to an intriguing links-style course that forces you to execute a host of shots you normally wouldn't even think to try — even if it is in New Jersey or Nebraska — don't feel guilty because you didn't get in a jet so you could hit similar shots in the more golf-pure environment of Britain or Ireland.

Go play as many as makes you happy. Go do it even though you may curse your luck in the pot bunkers and wonder why the waist-high fescue, which you would curse as a nuisance in your backyard, so colorfully frames the fairways with hues of gold in the summer and crimson in the fall.

It is irrelevant whether they are, in a way, facsimiles with borrowed traits. They are descendants of the first golf courses, and they give us a taste of a different style of golf. They are like a good Yuengling Porter, and when you have one near the brewery in eastern Pennsylvania, nobody wants to hear that the Yuengling isn't as good as a Guinness.

The proliferation of links-style courses in the United States probably traces its origin to the riveting 1991 Ryder Cup held on Pete and Alice Dye's nearly peerless Ocean Course at Kiawah Island. I've always thought Tiger Woods's victory in style at St. Andrews in 2000 did not hurt either.

Now, if you seek out the links-style courses nearby or far, you must know that it will require a unique set of golf skills. To name a few:

You must control the flight of the ball.

The trajectory of a shot is of paramount importance in windy conditions or on hard fairways, where a ball will run and run, often into a nasty bunker.

As my friend the golf pro Bryan Jones said, "You may have to learn to play a ground game and to choose a shorter club off the tee."

Jones taught for years next to the Ballyowen Golf Club in New Jersey, consistently selected as one of the best links-style public courses in the New York area.

"You may want to be shorter off the tee, because the shot must be placed to a strategically safe spot, not bombed with a driver," Bryan said.

In other words, high ball flight—the goal of many modern driver heads and modern golf balls—may not be your best friend on the links.

Watch your alignment.

Since there will be few, if any, trees or landmarks to guide you, it will be more difficult to aim.

Playing at St. Andrews several years ago, I was faced with this issue on one tee. Looking toward the water with nothing but a flat, vague stretch of ground in front of me, I asked my caddie where to aim.

"You see that cloud in the distance?" he said. "Aim at that, lad. And hurry up. It's moving."

Check your ego on the first, fescue-enveloped tee.

"I see amateur players trying the craziest, riskiest approach shots, like 220-yard carries over steep greenside bunkers," said Andy Bemis, the director of golf at the Tradition at Royal New Kent outside Williamsburg, Virginia, another popular links-style course.

"I tell people, 'Unless you think you can make that shot eight out of ten times, don't do it.' Admit to the reality of the situation and hit a 130-yard layup, because if you get in one of those 20-foot-deep bunkers, that's how a triple bogey gets on your card."

I can attest to this during a recent round at Royal New Kent, ranked sixteenth on *Golf Digest*'s list of the toughest golf courses in the country. I was in one bunker for so long, I am now expected to pay Virginia state income tax.

Whenever possible, putt the ball.

This is true even if you're 50 feet off the green.

"But you don't have to use your putter," Jones said. "That hybrid wood in your bag is a nice alternative for one of those long run-up shots across one of those large, open greens often seen on a links-style course."

When you are done with your links experience, you will remember the windswept views, the peculiar terrain, and the elevation changes. You will remember the blind shots and maybe a great shot out of a pot bunker. You may even take some wild fescue home with you wrapped around the hosel of your pitching wedge.

Chances are, you will not remember how many golf balls you lost. Or how high your score was. And that is as it should be.

"The first thing people usually say when they are done is 'Wow, that was hard,'" Bemis said. "The second thing they say is 'Wow, that was fun.'"

Playing a links-style course, wherever it may be, is a chance to see golf in a new light, and to do so with a respectful nod to the game's history. The course may not be entirely authentic. Does it matter? It shouldn't that day. Yes, try to get to St. Andrews and as many of the other iconic Scottish golf courses that time and budget allow. In the meantime, go have fun at a more accessible course with features designed in tribute to golf's ancestral roots.

6. Bizarre Golf Courses

Golf courses ought to be collected, but not as trophies. They should be collected for the stories you can tell afterward. Hence, everyone should try to play somewhere truly odd, quirky, or eccentric. Like where?

How about teeing it in northern Idaho where on the fourteenth hole you try to hit a movable, floating par-3 green? It's at the Coeur d'Alene Resort and the hole can play different distances since the whole green complex — a 15,000-square-foot putting surface, two bunkers, a few trees, and a dock — is perched in a lake. But the tee shot is usually about 150 yards. The green is then reached by a vessel called the Putter Boat. When you complete the hole — try to forget the age-old advice that all putts break toward a body of water — they give you a certificate noting your score. But you don't need the certificate. You have a story to tell for years to come instead.

Here is another example, which is more common than you would think. I played a golf course where you parked your car and visited the pro shop in the United States, but after the first tee shot you played eighteen holes in Canada.

Well, there were certain exceptions. If you hit it left off the tee on the first, second, or ninth hole, you would be chasing your ball back in the United States. At the open-to-the-public Aroostook Valley Country Club in northern Maine, there are a lot of unplanned border crossings. And each time you cross the border, the time changes as well.

How often do you get to hit your golf ball so far it goes back in time? Now, that's a story.

The locals say the entire golf course, clubhouse, pro shop, and parking lot were originally thought to be laid out in Canada in the early 1920s when it opened. Subsequent surveying repositioned some of the property in the United States. Everyone is pretty casual about the situation. There are no border guards or customs officials inspecting golf bags as they weave back and forth from country to country.

There are other golf courses on national borders. The Green Zone Golf Club has nine holes in Finland and nine holes in Sweden. In the summer, the sun also never goes down. So you can tee off at 2:00 a.m. and seemingly defect to another country. Now, that's a golf story.

If you go to Scandinavia for golf, you might as well stop at Greenland along the way. There you can play a golf course laid out on icebergs and fjords near Uummannaq. They hold the World Ice Golf Championships there. The holes are a little shorter because the extreme cold makes the ball travel less far (the golfers aren't too limber either). The holes cut in the ice, however, are larger than normal. The ball is orange and the greens, like most everything else, are white.

For the opposite extreme, there is the lowest and perhaps hottest golf course in Death Valley, California. At 218 feet below sea level, summer temperatures can exceed 130 degrees at the Devil's Golf Course, where they like to say, "Only the Devil can shoot par." Now, there's a challenge a serious golfer cannot pass up.

You can play golf inside the Indianapolis Motor Speedway, site of the Indy 500, when you pay the greens fees at Brickyard Crossing. Four holes loop inside the grounds of the historic speedway — routed counterclockwise by the iconoclastic course designer, the onetime Indianapolis insurance salesman Pete Dye.

You can go to Oahu in Hawaii and play what may be the hardest golf course in America, the Koolau Golf Club, which measures more than 7,300 yards built entirely in a rainforest. A trip around Koolau's eighteen holes means passing through three climate zones, past stunning waterfalls, and weathering extreme, dramatic elevation changes. Officials there keep not only the course record (62) but the record for most balls lost in eighteen holes (59). Now, there's a record made to be broken.

Those are some of the exotic choices to pique your imagination. But you need not go to Death Valley, Hawaii, or Greenland to find odd and quirky places to knock around a little white golf ball. Within fifty miles of home, the chances are good there is a golf course built out of a former quarry, laid out across a desert, or built across a capped garbage dump. Golf sprouts in all kinds of bizarre places.

A golf course where the bunkers are filled with a strange black soot or ground-up seashells — I have seen both — is out there waiting to be found. There are courses where the greens are oil-covered sand. There are golf courses where only the greens and tees are real grass and the fairways and rough are artificial turf. There are golf courses illuminated by lights so night play is possible, which is a real treat for those of us whose circadian rhythm falls in the realm of the night owl. There are golf courses where the wildlife is not a sidelight but in play, as in "Don't hit it right of fairway; that's where the snakes and alligators are." There are courses where power lines are in play, crisscrossing multiple fairways. This being golf, only well-struck shots seem to ever strike the power lines. The wayward shots that you pray some force field will strike down never hit the power lines.

There are golf courses with peculiar rock formations, sinkholes, and burned-out automobiles in the middle of the fairways. In an attempt at insurance fraud a few years ago, a golf course owner in Texas buried an aging tractor in one of his fairways, then reported it stolen. The tractor, of course, surfaced after a particularly relentless rainstorm. Golfers had to play around it for most of one summer.

There are gimmick golf courses, like the Tour 18 courses, which attempt to replicate famous golf holes from around the country, or the world, packaged into one eighteen-hole arrangement. In other words, they re-create Amen Corner from Augusta National and the eighteenth hole from Pebble Beach. The first hole of a Tour 18 might be the eighteenth hole at Harbor Town. When you play these courses, do you really feel as if you're at Augusta National, then Pebble Beach, and then TPC Sawgrass?

No, of course not. When I played the Tour 18 course in Houston, I knew I had never left Texas since they weren't, for example, able to re-create the 150-foot and centuries-old loblolly pines from Augusta National. There was obviously no Pacific Ocean waiting off the tee of the replica eighteenth hole from Pebble Beach either. But they got the distances right, and you could still see how you would play the short twelfth hole at Augusta National. You could replicate shots you've seen on television.

The point is, it was something different. It was golf that shook me out of my routine. And I brought home some more golf stories, and they are far more valuable than any trophies.

7. The Best Municipal Golf Course in Your County or State

The humble local muni is the heart and pulse of golf around the world. More than 80 percent of all golf is played on public golf courses, something overlooked in most every conversation about important golf courses. Important golf courses are ones where you see this scene:

Within a short walk of the clubhouse, pro shop, or small starter's shack, the stalls in a parking lot fill up one by one. Golfers emerge quickly and trunks immediately pop open. And beside those trunks, in a chorus line of sorts, golfers perform that inimitable dance: the one-legged, putting-on-the-golf-shoe hop.

It is as funny as it is soothing. There are a lot of mores in golf, and this custom is not appropriate in every setting. But here, it is a welcome sight.

There has been much hand-wringing lately about a decline in the number of golf rounds played in America. And indeed, some high-end golf clubs and resorts are doggedly in pursuit of the recreational golfer who doesn't seem to have the free time to hang around the country club the way the golfers of a generation ago did. But the affordable, quality municipal golf courses are alive and well.

The reasons are obvious: They are affordable and unpretentious. They give people what they most want — a chance to play and to exercise outside at a good value. Their fairways are full of people happily tugging on their pull carts.

The average cost of the average round of golf in the United States is $22 and $36 with a golf cart. That is because of the local muni, which has made golf more open to more people than ever before.

There is no secret to their success. They are fun to play and they do some smart things to keep the crowds moving. The golf hazards, for example, are penal but generally not treacherous. If you hit a ball into the woods, you will probably find it and have a way out of trouble.

"We make sure the woods are more sparse and not dense," James Stewart, the head PGA professional at the popular Blue Hill Golf Course in Orangeburg, New York, said. "And we manicure the areas under the trees so the rough is not too high. It helps the speed of play.

We don't want people having to spend too much time looking for the ball or trying to figure out how to get out of the woods."

Blue Hill does, on average, 70,000 rounds a year, twice the national average for a public course. That's a healthy business. Many municipal courses are busy for good reason; in many locales, they may be the best course for many miles around.

Yes, they can be crowded. Some can be hard to get on, requiring some very advance planning, or skullduggery, to obtain a choice tee time. But in most places there is a local muni that serves the public well without too much hassle, and that is the golf course you should visit semi-regularly — even if you belong to a private club.

It will restore your belief in golf. Muni golf is a refresher course in what gives the game its appeal. Because golf is not really about the makeup of the sand in the bunkers or the Stimpmeter reading of the greens. It's about getting the ball in the hole and trying to do it with a bunch of other people inspired by the same goal. When finished, you sit back in a restful bar, probably with a window onto the final green, so you can watch others trying to do the same thing.

And through that window you will also see something else: the one-legged parking-lot hop. By the way, when you visit that local muni, you can change your shoes in the locker room or restroom if you like. It's perfectly acceptable.

But your legs — and your sense of humor — won't be warmed up when you stand on the first tee.

8. Golf Courses in Hard-to-Find Places

Why work so hard, you say? I've been preaching that good golf is where you find it. And it's true. Ever looked out the window of a jet? There are golf courses everywhere. But going the extra mile — and maybe another 300 miles after that — leads to the most remarkable surprises. It's another step in getting out of your routine. Finding golf where you don't expect it is part of being a real golfer, too.

So, that's how I ended up in Nova Scotia. One weekend I started dreaming of playing again in Scotland. But all I had available was a long weekend. And my budget was relatively small, too. And that brought me to new Scotland — Nova Scotia, one of the Canadian Maritime Provinces.

Golf in Nova Scotia does not replicate golf in Scotland. But here are some of the province's distinguishing advantages: It is unspoiled and has about 5,000 miles of seacoast, some of it lined with spectacular golf courses. And you will never have to pretend you have left the United States. You will know it in dozens of ways, from the accents of a friendly host populace — a mix of Scottish, Acadian, English, and native Mi'kmaq people — to the moose and bald eagles that frequent the golf layouts the way cart girls do at resorts in the United States.

Several courses in Nova Scotia have a Scottish coastal feel, but there are other appealing characteristics, chief among them a pristine environment lightly visited by traveling golfers. What you find in Nova Scotia, which is reachable by car, jet, or ferry, are public courses with striking sea views that get about one-tenth of the play of many United States golf courses.

Lodging is ample, Nova Scotia's cultural history is preserved and engaging, and the dining choices — particularly when it comes to lobster, mussels, and scallops — are plentiful. Hop on a morning flight to Halifax and by the afternoon, you could be standing on the fourth tee at the beautiful oceanside Northumberland Links, where if you tripped backward, you would nearly fall into the picturesque blue water of the Northumberland Strait.

Behind the green are the remains of a scuttled wooden boat, part of the hole's design. In this majestic setting, water is visible from nearly every hole, as are Prince Edward Island and the Gulf of St. Lawrence beyond.

A few minutes down the road from homey Northumberland is a dazzling golfing and lodging choice, the exclusive Fox Harb'r Golf Resort and Spa, voted the best new course in Canada by *Golf Digest* when it opened in 2001. Fox Harb'r is exclusive and pricey, with 1,100 gated acres that include not only championship golf but also a private beach, fly-fishing ponds, manor-style townhouses, fine dining, and an airstrip.

A four-hour drive to the northeast, and light-years away in atmosphere, is the Nova Scotia island of Cape Breton, where I was preparing to hit from the edge of a fairway one afternoon late one August when a ten-foot bull moose walked up and asked to play through.

Actually, moose, at 1,200 pounds, don't ask permission to do anything. But this one apparently liked golf. In fact, a minute after he quietly arrived, he meandered into the woods and watched me hit my shot from about 40 feet away.

This, I discovered, will quicken even a lengthy pre-shot routine. Perhaps that's why there is no slow-play epidemic in Nova Scotia. Or it could be that players do not want to waste time waggling a club when they could be taking in the views, the wildlife, and the peaceful landscape.

My moose encounter was at Highlands Links, an intriguing if occasionally raw course designed in 1939 by the Scottish-influenced Stanley Thompson. It has been rated one of the world's top one hundred layouts by *Golf Magazine* and is in Cape Breton Highlands National Park, a spectacular public playground spread across cliffs above the ocean.

While there, stay at the Keltic Lodge, where doormen in kilts will greet you. Eat some delectable crab for dinner and attend a ceilidh, a traditional Gaelic music-and-dance social gathering. In the morning, stroll over for a tidy three-and-a-half-hour round of golf.

You may not be in Scotland, but you will undoubtedly know you are not back home.

And that's the point of these extra-effort golf excursions.

Revelations are everywhere, and it doesn't require leaving the country to find them. About 1,500 miles south of Nova Scotia is the Old World golf spot, the Greenbrier Resort in White Sulphur Springs, West Virginia. Go there to channel the ghost of Sam Snead, who called the Greenbrier home for more than sixty years. The Greenbrier is not easy to reach, but people have been doing it since 1778. That has included pro golfers. The PGA Tour has made the Greenbrier a regular stop for decades.

There are many golf spots well off the interstate highways. Consider, for example, the Links of North Dakota, near the Canadian border in northwest North Dakota. It's been called the best out-of-the-way golf course in America. Driving to the course is an adventure, with the final thirty minutes usually in solitude without another car in sight. It is a stark, links-style layout designed by Stephen Kay with sweeping views of the desolate plains and Lake Sakakawea. It is one of the eighteen golf courses that make up the Lewis and Clark Golf Trail, and after ten shots you will know you are in neither the Midwest nor western Canada. This is the land Lewis and Clark mapped with their Corps of Discovery. Go play golf at the Links of North Dakota and discovery is indeed the likely outcome.

Not too far from where the Lewis and Clark expedition reached the Pacific Ocean is the Bandon Dunes Resort, another hard-to-reach place that golfers are nevertheless finding in droves. So if the four golf courses at Bandon Dunes are far from unknown, they still demand a visit. They are more than a clichéd destination. On the shoreline of southern Oregon, the courses have been built on rugged, windswept land. The elements change with unpredictable weather patterns, and because of that, so does the golf you are playing. It is natural, with huge dunes and towering pines, and it is an unforgettable golf experience.

Sometimes the rarest finds are near prominent golf places but nonetheless off the beaten track. That would describe the Tobacco Road Golf Club, which is not far from Pinehurst, the North Carolina golf hub. Tobacco Road is one of the brilliant designs from the underrated golf architect Mike Strantz, who was on his way to becoming a foremost American golf architect until he died of cancer at the age of fifty. Strantz's Tobacco Road is an hour's drive from Pinehurst and probably gets one-tenth the visits from recreational golfers. Driving there, you would certainly not expect anything special. And that's the best part.

After you check your map or GPS two or three times to make sure you are going the right way, Tobacco Road will appear on the horizon. You will still think you're in the middle of nowhere. And indeed, Tobacco Road was built out of a wasteland. But the inventive Strantz, who had a side career as an artist and painter, saw the wasteland as a canvas. And he built near-mountains on it. Each hole offers new and different challenges. One fairway might be a mighty, welcoming 100 yards wide, the next one no more than 30 yards wide. The greens have strange, abnormal dimensions and shapes. One looks like a giant smile, 80 feet deep at the middle and only 15 feet deep at its narrowest points.

You've got to find your way to a golf course like that. These kinds of golf surprises are everywhere. The essential point is that great golf is not always easy to find. Moreover, some of the most unanticipated delights are decidedly hidden. That sounds like a metaphor for life, so why should golf — sport's ultimate parable for life — be any different?

Go the extra mile. Find golf where, it seems, nothing belongs. You will likely make other discoveries in the guise of a golf trip.

9. Golf Wherever You Are

I have a policy: Some of the best golf is played in places you never thought you would be. Here's what I mean by that.

It means always keep your clubs in your trunk, and wherever you are, see if there is a golf course around the next corner. Because the golf course around the corner — the one you did not expect to visit — is always, at that moment, the greatest golf course in the world. Golf you never expected to play is always the greatest golf in the world.

There are a number of ways to make sure you find these golf courses. Going away for the weekend for a wedding? Get out and play at least nine holes. There will be a course around the corner.

Niece's graduation? Plenty of time for a quick nine before the ceremony.

High school reunion? Perfect for a long golf outing with your old pals.

Going to the in-laws'? Definitely get out of the house and find a golf course somewhere. Better yet, sneak out so you're alone.

Baptisms, bar mitzvahs, anniversaries, even Tupperware parties — all are excuses to find a golf course around the corner.

There are variations to the theme. Fourth of July barbecues are a great time to get a chipping contest started in the backyard. Helping someone move? Who doesn't want to roll some putts across the carpet of the new house? It's the best way to check if the floors are level.

One of the great things about golf is that it is everywhere in America. You can't say that about too many things if you think about it. But it is a fact that you can find some kind of golf course near every American city or isolated town, and everywhere in between.

Where should we play golf? The best answer might be to play wherever we are. It may be the best way to get to know the area and the people who live there. You will learn about golf in all its forms.

Finding hidden gems — places you never expected to play — conveys an air of discovery. Surprised at your good fortune to find a golf course around the corner, you get out of the car feeling as if you have been handed an unforeseen gift. And the gift is the chance to play golf on a new, or old, golf course that will likely bring surprises around every bend. Relaxing enough to let golf surprise you is one of the game's purest joys.

That golf experience is out there waiting for you. It's probably right around the corner, wherever you are. And you will never forget it.

There is nothing routine about that.

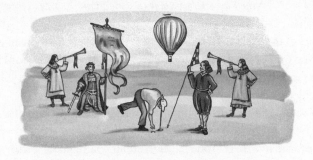

14

Golf's Holy Grail

Holes in One and What They Teach Us

A hole in one is amazing when you think of the different
universes this white mass of molecules has to pass
through on its way to the hole.

MAC O'GRADY, golf teacher/guru and former Tour player

A 102-YEAR-OLD woman has had a hole in one. So has a 101-year-old man. Children as young as 5 years old have had holes in one. Phil Mickelson had his first when he was 8. Tiger Woods when he was 6. Michelle Wie when she was 12. Golfers who fell down while swinging the club have still struck the ball and had it go in the hole from the tee. People have broken their club, or had it fly out of their hands, and still had the ball find the hole. People get holes in one after their tee shots have hit trees, maintenance vehicles, sprinkler heads, bunker rakes, even a bird in flight.

One-armed golfers have had holes in one. So have double leg amputees. A bunch of golfers have had a hole in one while golfing right-handed and then had another hole in one later in life while golfing left-handed. In 2010, a woman in Tampa, Florida, hit a hole in one with her first swing on the first hole she had ever played.

People have had holes in one on 500-yard par 5s, and on hundreds of par 4s. Some professional golfers, during their careers, have had fifty or more holes in one. Leo Fiyalko, who is legally blind and ninety-two years old, made a hole in one.

"I was just trying to put the ball on the green," said Fiyalko, who hit a 5-iron from 110 yards.

Performers have had holes in one (Frank Sinatra, Smokey Robinson, and Justin Timberlake), as have star athletes from other sports (Roger Clemens and John Elway). And so have presidents (Dwight Eisenhower, Gerald Ford, and Richard Nixon). Nixon called his ace "the greatest thrill of my life." Then again, it was 1961.

There are as many as 150,000 holes in one every year in the United States, and 20 holes in one, on average, every hour somewhere in the world.

If that makes you feel as if every golfer should have made a hole in one by now — and if, like me, you haven't had one — consider this: The odds of an average recreational player making a hole in one are 12,000 to 1. If you're playing a 200-yard par 3, the odds are 150,000 to 1.

But the hole in one is a very powerful concept in golf. The phenomenon of the hole in one is a window into golf itself. It is a shot that inherently encapsulates all of the game's authentic and ethereal elements. It is happenstance and ultimate precision at once. It is egalitarian and exclusive at once. It is a shot launched against long odds, landed with innocent hope, and finished with an exclamation of unsurpassable perfection. At that moment, in that place, no golfer on Earth can hit a better shot. The hole in one is the only time a golfer truly succeeds at golf. (Well, for one hole.)

It is an accomplishment of a career, the embodiment of the golfing spirit, a fleeting moment to cherish forevermore. It is the essence of golf in a second, and at the same time, it is a career achievement in a lifetime sport. It's a hole in one and there is nothing quite like it in any other sport.

"Average people cannot wake up tomorrow and expect to have the chance to do something perfectly in sports, like whiff Alex Rodriguez with three pitches," said Chris Rodell, author of the 2003 book *Hole in One!*

"But the average person could one day hit a golf shot that Bobby

Jones, Ben Hogan, Jack Nicklaus, or Tiger Woods could not do better. When you make a hole in one, in that moment that is the greatest shot ever."

Have you ever asked someone about the hole in one he or she made? People describe it like they are describing the birth of a child. It's more than an achievement; it is almost celestial.

Consider Annika Sorenstam, who has had three career aces. She is one of the greatest golfers in history with sixty-seven professional tournament victories. But ask her about holes in one, and what she recalls is that her sister, Charlotta, winner of exactly one pro tournament, has had nine holes in one.

"That's three times your total, Sis," Charlotta said once on a practice range as she stood alongside her sister.

"I know, I know," Annika answered. "Don't rub it in."

I told you this hole-in-one thing was powerful.

Not surprisingly, the golf world has spent a lot of time studying the hole in one. Dr. Francis J. Scheid, the former chairman of the mathematics department at Boston University, was known until his death in 2011 as Professor Golf. He lived to be ninety years old and did calculations on the 2 billion golf shots launched into the skies above par-3 holes every year in the United States alone.

Among the things he learned:

A Tour player has a 1-in-3,000 chance of making a hole in one. For someone with a golf handicap of 5 or lower, the odds are 1 in 6,000. An average golfer needs on average about 3,000 rounds of golf to make a hole in one. A better player, on average, should make a hole in one in 1,250 rounds.

The chances that two players in one foursome will make holes in one in the same round are 1 in 17 million. The chances even a low handicapper has of making two holes in one in the same round are 1 in 67 million. That hasn't prevented it from happening.

Sanjay Kuttemperoor of Naples, Florida, did it in 2006 while playing a round in Michigan. And yes, it was witnessed. The renowned instructor Rick Smith happened to be in Kuttemperoor's group. But get this: Kuttemperoor said he had never even had a birdie before that round.

In less than two hours during the second round of the 1989 U.S. Open, Doug Weaver, Mark Wiebe, Jerry Pate, and Nick Price each aced the 167-yard sixth hole at the Oak Hill Country Club outside Rochester. The odds against four professionals achieving such a record in a field of 156 were estimated to be 1.89 quadrillion to 1.

Some other hole-in-one data:

- Average age of hole-in-one golfer: 44.7
- Gender: 84 percent male
- Average yardage of hole: 150.5
- Club used most in making an ace: 7-iron
- Day of the week most aces occur: Friday
- Day of the week fewest aces occur: Sunday
- Ball used the most: Titleist

Dr. Scheid was not the only one with hole-in-one expertise. Various companies provide hole-in-one insurance to golf tournaments sponsoring hole-in-one prize contests. They say that in a typical golf outing with 100 amateurs and four par 3s on the course, there is about a 1-in-32 chance someone will make a hole in one.

The fact is, crummy golfers make aces all the time.

"We have to verify every claim before we pay the prize," said Greg Esterhai, co-owner of US Hole in One, a company that provides hole-in-one insurance to about 8,000 events annually. "About half the time, it's a good golfer who says, 'Ho-hum, just won another Cadillac.' But the other half of the time, when we ask about the shot, they say: 'It was horrendous — barely in the air. It bounced off the cart path three times.'"

Olympic ski racer Lindsey Vonn had a hole in one four months after she won a gold medal at the 2010 Vancouver Olympics. It was her second time playing eighteen holes. And she never saw it go in.

"It was a scramble and the other three players had already shanked their balls in the woods," Vonn said, recounting her shot at the 167-yard par 3 at a course in Monterey, California. "I was last to hit, and when I saw the ball sailing toward the green, I was happy we were going to have a ball in play."

She did not continue to watch the ball. Instead, she bent over to pick up her tee.

"All of a sudden everyone started yelling and freaking out," Vonn said. "I never saw it go in and I didn't believe them until we got to the green and I picked it out of the hole."

I've had some personal experience with holes in one, even though I have not made one. I was playing in Orlando in the 1990s, and when you paid for your round they gave you a little key card, like the kind used to open hotel doors. When you got to the tee of the first par 3 in the round, you used the card to activate a video camera that captured your shot from tee to green. If you made a hole in one, you won $5,000.

A married couple was playing in front of me and since I was playing alone, after a couple of holes they invited me to join them. The husband was a decent player, but the wife looked as if she had played golf maybe once or twice before.

At the first prizewinning par 3, no one got close to making an ace. But at the next par 3, the husband hit a shot that bounced twice and rolled into the hole.

He jumped in the air with his club over his head and screamed. So did his wife, except she screamed: "You jerk, why didn't you do that before? We could have won $5,000!"

I had to hit after him. It was a hard act to follow.

The hole-in-one phenomenon can undoubtedly be as peculiar and vexing as the rest of golf. And sometimes, just as unfair.

Take the story of John Murphy, who made a hole in one in 1982 on the 175-yard fifth hole at the Wil-Mar Golf Club in Raleigh, North Carolina. As Rodell wrote in his book, Murphy was playing alone and no one witnessed the shot, so he knew his ace would forever be unofficial. When Murphy was done with his round, he went to the clubhouse and told a friend about his fate. The two went back out to the fifth hole so Murphy could better recount what happened. He teed another ball, swung, and put that shot in the hole.

That doesn't count officially either. A hole in one must occur during a round of play, and in most cases, the round must be completed.

Two holes in one in the same day and neither counted. Is this where Murphy's law came from?

But just the prospect and proximity to a hole in one can have a certain charm, too, much like the rest of golf. The closest I have ever come to a hole in one was during a round I played with my daughters several years ago. On a 140-yard hole, my tee shot hit the lip of the hole on the fly, spun around the hole, smacked the flagstick, and settled an inch from the cup.

Standing next to me, my daughter Elise, who was then five, turned and said: "That was so cool, Dad. Do it again."

What do these stories tell us? What do they mean?

I'll offer one more story that might be enlightening. More than a decade ago, I was playing in Arizona with a sportswriter colleague. My friend wasn't a strong player, and that day he was playing very poorly. We had played the day before as well, when he must have shot 115. And not a good 115 either.

My friend is a good athlete and he had been playing golf for at least five years, but he could not grasp the game in all its intricacies. He was at war with golf, and there is a long casualty list in that pitched battle. My friend would fix his full swing, then lose all his touch on the greens. He would fix his short game and instead start spraying everything off the tee.

It was not working out, and as we played that day he was talking about giving up golf for good. He sounded as if he meant it.

Then, on the twelfth hole, from an elevated tee that framed the green like a Broadway stage, he hit a pure 5-iron that bounced on the front of the green, skipped 8 feet forward, and rolled another 10 feet right into the hole. He whooped and danced, high-fived everyone in sight, bought drinks, made phone calls, and spent the rest of the day—the rest of weekend—with his feet seemingly never touching the ground. We all started calling him "Ace," and he kept the stupidest, happiest smile on his face for many hours.

At the same time, some sort of cosmic golf button had been pushed. My friend not only did not give up golf—how could he?—he slowly became a better and better golfer. I'm not saying it was entirely because of the hole in one. Practicing more and taking lessons certainly helped, but the hole in one changed his relationship with the game.

In that singular uniquely inspiring moment, my friend became a golfer instead of someone who plays golf.

Similar transformations happen on golf courses all over the world every day, and not just after making a hole in one. It happens when someone is playing alone and makes two consecutive birdies for the first time, then smiles a knowing smile of triumph and does not care that no one was there to see it. The realization and the satisfaction are internal.

It happens when you hit your ball in the woods during a match, go look for it, and happily come upon a ball sitting up near a clearing with a view of the green. But when you bend over to inspect the ball, you see it isn't yours. And though no one but you would have ever known that wasn't your ball, you keep looking. When your ball is found behind a tree trunk, you feel a little wounded, but you know a golfer has to play it where it lies.

It happens when you remind a partner about a wedge left on the fringe of the green. It happens when you find something positive to say after someone else's bad shot, and it happens when you are having a bad day but keep your good humor, grinning instead of groaning to avoid casting a pall on the whole foursome.

It happens when you find yourself jittery on the first tee but calm yourself with a trick or two — like throwing a ball a few inches in the air, then catching it with your hand. Besides, you say to yourself, the first shot is just that. It's only the first shot. Golf is a lifetime journey of golf shots.

It happens when you flawlessly chip or float a shot over a greenside bunker, channeling the tips you read from Butch Harmon or Annika Sorenstam. It happens when you ignore the water in front of a green and send your approach shot soaring to the safe part of the green. As you walk confidently toward your ball, you think, "What water?"

It happens when you catch yourself calling a puddle "casual water" or when you realize you haven't said "sand trap" or "pin" in a year because you know it is always a "bunker" and always the "flagstick." You feel silly and a bit stilted for adopting the language of golf as your own, but you cannot help it; the terms tumble out of your mouth without affectation. You are a golfer.

And speaking of language, when someone asks if you want to play Bingo, Bango, Bongo, you knowingly ask for the scorecard to keep track of the many points on every green. When it is suggested that a partner's drive had a certain Linda Ronstadt quality to it, you do not break into song. You know that your partner Blue Bayou, and there is something oddly funny in that. On the other hand, it pains you to put a Bo Derek on your scorecard. But you do write down a 10.

It happens when every shot is going sideways, but you do not say the S-word. You recall that "it" has afflicted the very best golfers of all time. They survived. Every golfer survives that malady, that unspeakable terror. Eventually.

Eventually? Isn't that what one of your caddies said when you asked if you could get to the green with a 4-iron? Eventually, indeed.

It happens on a quiet, cool evening on an empty nine-hole golf course next to the foot of a mountain or beside a river or bordering a valley lit by a sunset. It happens when you realize golf brought you to this vista. The game is one shot at a time, and at that moment, the next shot is all that matters, and yet it does not matter at all. Because there is always a next shot.

It happens when something amazingly ridiculous occurs — a shot that ricochets off the smallest tree branch to bounce on a cart path where it deflects off a golf cart only to bounce into a drainage gully that sends your golf ball trundling 25 yards backward where it plops into a small murky pond.

You will look at your partners and they will look at you. You will laugh. They will laugh. You will shrug your shoulders at such a preposterous outcome in an athletic event that is supposed to be ruled by basic physics but somehow seems beyond it. Only in golf. And only fully understood by golfers.

I would instinctively rub the long-since-healed red welt on my forehead.

This is the journey golfers have chosen. This is where we go together, down the road with our hopes as a defense against certain disappointment and our fears as ballast against unexpected delight. To be a golfer means finding perseverance in stores we never knew we had. It means carrying a bag of fourteen clubs, each designed to hit the golf ball a certain distance, even though none of them truly manage the most pivotal distance in golf—the 5 inches between your ears.

To be a golfer means understanding that surprise will be common. It means that good, even spectacular, golf shots will occur like out-of-body experiences. It means engaging in a curious oneness with nature as you ponder every new technological advance to get an advantage. It means conforming to centuries-old group protocols while playing a game where no one but you decides what you hit, when you hit, or where you hit it. It means being assigned the simple act of tapping a small white ball 2 feet into a little hole and sensing certain failure beforehand. It means hitting a small white ball 170 yards off a tee toward a little hole and believing that one day your shot will result in the perfect outcome.

And perhaps that's the power of the hole in one. It is the result of faith and a belief that anything can happen. Emboldened by that notion, the golf tribe marches forward in spite of the odds, maybe even because of the odds. The hole in one and other revelations are out there to be found, conquests to trump the greatest odds.

Have you ever noticed that when someone makes a hole in one, everyone celebrates? Your opponents rejoice, caddies yelp, anyone watching howls. The responses are automatic, inherent, and intuitive. The celebration lifts everyone as if we all had something to do with the shot. And truth be told, we did. We are all in this together. Feeling abandoned by golf is a frequent emotion, but in time, you learn that golfers never walk alone. We survive together.

Golfers are always in step, bound by the game's mysteries like a secret covenant. That's why golfers at parties assemble in circles spontaneously even if they arrived as strangers. There is a tacit harmony. Individual golf shots may break you down but the game always unites. The shared journey is everlasting. So a hole in one becomes everyone's achievement because, for that moment, we won. It went in. The golf gods smiled but not as much as we will.

I've even heard people say afterward, "That wasn't so hard." Which almost makes sense. Sure, after all, that is where you were aiming.

The tribe would nod. We would walk to the next hole thinking, "Let's do that again." You never know.

It is golf.

March on.

Acknowledgments

I am fortunate to have had hundreds of assists and acts of generosity in getting this book completed. That probably goes all the way back to the guy behind the counter of the pitch and putt near my house in Connecticut who let me play my very first real golf even though I had only three quarters in my pocket that day (nine holes cost a dollar). Of course, it turned out to be a good marketing ploy. I liked it so much I dragged all my grammar-school friends to that pitch and putt for the rest of the summer.

Speaking of marketing, this book wouldn't have happened without the encouragement, counsel, and insight of my agent, Scott Waxman. Much more than a fan of the "On Par" columns, he saw how much further we could take the conversation with recreational golfers.

Picking up where Scott left off, my editor, Susan Canavan, had a clear vision of the manuscript well before I started typing in earnest. With humor and faith she pushed for every little improvement but never seemed pushy. She also knows how to read writers as well as writing—a peerless skill.

At the *New York Times* so many people have made the *On Par* golf package find a footing and prosper, including Joe Sexton, Tom Jolly, Dave Anderson, Sandy Keenan, Patty La Duca, Tom Connelly, Jason Stallman, Mike Abrams, Lee Yarosh, Naila-Jean Meyers, Ann Derry, Matt Orr, Rich Tanner, Dave Frank, Kassie Bracken, Stephen Hirsch, Larry Dorman, and Alex Ward.

At the United States Golf Association, my thanks to Bernie Loehr for his endless patience in explaining the Rules of Golf. Dick Rugge has done much the same for equipment regulations.

My friend the PGA pro Bryan Jones has cared so much about *On Par* he has been willing to stand with me in the hot, glaring sun for scores of hours as we made more than fifty videos. His humor and golf erudition — an impressive combination — contributed to whole sections of the book and made it better. Thanks also to Adam Donlin at the Ballyowen Golf Club and Art Walton at the Crystal Springs Resort.

My former colleague and frequent golf companion Mike Celizic, who died of cancer while this book was being written, taught me much about the game and what makes it special. I will always miss not being able to play with him.

And finally, besides listening to all my meanderings about golf for decades, my wife, Joyce, also did considerable research before I wrote a word of the manuscript. And where Joyce left off my daughter Anne D. seamlessly picked up the research. Chronologically next but hardly second, my daughter Elise suggested the book's subtitle. My youngest, Jack, has the benefit of extra years of my parental wisdom. Surprisingly, he puts in more regular time on the golf course with me than anyone else in the family. That helps my handicap. I have become his.

All three kids put up with the countless times I would be practicing my swing in front of their high chair — using their baby spoon as a substitute for a club. Don't worry, I fed them eventually. My wife has let me putt back and forth in the living room for more than twenty years. In general, no one has yelped — well, not too much — when I would snatch away the clicker to change the TV channel to some golf tournament.

"Not golf again," someone might squeal.

"What? They're coming down the eighteenth fairway of the Phoenix Open," I would say.

"Yeah, and it's also time for the Super Bowl kickoff."

"Oh, that," I would answer. "They play that every year."

What a game.

Index